For many years now, Henry Cooper has been one of the most popular of national figures – for his courage, his skill, his modesty and his humour.

He was the first person to put Muhammad Ali (then Cassius Clay) down in professional boxing. He was for many years British, Commonwealth and European heavyweight champion. He was twice voted BBC TV Sports Personality of the year.

At 47, Henry Cooper feels as fit as he did at 27 – despite having retired from professional boxing.

Get Fit For Life

HENRY COOPER

SPHERE BOOKS LIMITED
30-32 Gray's Inn Road, London WC1X 8JL

First published in Great Britain by Sphere Books Ltd 1982
Copyright © Henry Cooper, Victorama Limited
and the Health Education Council

Set in Lasercomp Times

Printed and bound in Great Britain by
©ollins, Glasgow

Much of the information and material in this book is based directly on the work of the Health Education Council and is reproduced by kind permission. While every effort has been made to ensure the accuracy of all the material used, the Health Education Council can take no responsibility for the book as a whole and is in no way associated with the publication beyond the advice given. Grateful acknowledgement for their kind co-operation is also due to the Sports Council, and to Dr Alan Maryon-Davis, Acting Chief Medical Officer of the Health Education Council, Jane Thomas of Queen Elizabeth College, London, Dr Ben Hamilton and Dr Heather Montrose.

CONTENTS

Introduction

How fit are you? I don't mean super-humanly fit with a physique like a Greek god, but fit to tackle the problems of everyday life. Without wishing to sound boastful or vain, I am proud to say that I still feel just as fit as I did twenty years ago. I still do the same things and certainly don't feel any older, and I hope that in twenty years' time I'll still be just as fit.

So, how fit are you? Do you get out of breath running for the bus? Are you tired and irritable at the end of a long day? Can you still touch your toes, or has your tummy grown so big that you can't even see your feet?.

By the time you've finished with this book you'll not only be fit enough to run after the bus, but so fit that you'll be able to dispense with it altogether!

Every one of us has the gift of a body, and the very precious gift of a life in front of us to put that body to good use. I think we owe it to ourselves to look after that body and make the very most of the life we have. Not everyone can achieve fame or fortune, but everyone has a right to fitness, and nothing can take the place of good health. Whatever your age or condition this book will show you how you can use your time and energy to the best advantage, so that when you wake up in the morning you will not only feel fit for work, but on top form to enjoy every moment of the day.

Without being too technical or highfalutin', I have tried to look at all aspects of our everyday lives and the ways in which we can make the most of what we have, and so be in the very best physical and psychological state. Feeling fit isn't simply the state that your body is in, but your mind as well.

You will discover that keeping fit doesn't have to be a

chore. It doesn't mean exercising daily for hours so that you feel worn out, or living on carrot juice and lettuce leaves. Neither does it mean changing your lifestyle nor routine to keep fit. The object is to be fit for the life you lead, so I've tried to suggest ways in which you can maximise your time and exercise whilst vacuuming the lounge, or dictating a letter to your secretary, flying around the world, or simply lying flat on your back in bed. Whether you're in the big world of high finance or a housebound housewife, you have a perfect right to good health.

I hope you will discover that this book is not just another boring lecture on physical exercise, telling you all the things you shouldn't do, you've heard that all before – instead it is a practical guide to a new and healthier you. Use it as a handbook to advise you on everything from eating to exercising, from sport to sleep, from posture to plastic surgery. Let it be your secret to a new life, for you and your whole family. Make yourself not only fit for life, but live a longer life too, and let your great-grandchildren in on the secret!

Here you will find all you need to make you feel good . . . all over!

HENRY COOPER

Chapter One

What Does It Mean To Be Fit and How Fit Are You?

Most of us like to think that we are fit. We may have a few aches and pains here and there, but unless we have a specific illness and need to go to the doctor then we must be in good health . . . mustn't we? OK, we puff a bit when running for the bus, and touching our toes is a bit of a strain, and we don't sleep quite as well as we used to – but surely everyone is like that? Basically we're fit as a fiddle. Or so we think . . .

Fitness is one of the most misused words in the English language. When the average person says he feels 'fit', he may mean anything from a vague feeling of well-being as he takes a deep breath of fresh air by an open window, to a sensation of comfort while taking severe exercise which would make an untrained man stiff for a week. The Sports Council uses the term 'physical fitness' to mean the capacity to enjoy moderate endurance activity, such as walking, cycling or jogging, appropriate to the person's age, without discomfort either during or after exercise. If we are able to live an active life and work and play as we wish, we generally feel that we are getting all the exercise we need.

So why bother to exercise? If you're fit enough to drive a car, use a washing machine, work the motor mower or the electric drill, that's all that matters isn't it? The truth is – No.

We tend to forget that in our everyday lives, however much we move around, there are parts of our body and certain muscles that we use far less than the rest. As a result, some of our muscles become weak, soft and flabby, instead of firm and strong. Perhaps while carrying the shopping home, or a heavy briefcase to work, you will always use your right hand. In time the muscles of that arm will be much stronger than the left and eventually your body will compensate for the weight by causing the body to lean to one side, the result being rounded shoulders and bad posture.

Although we live in a highly technological world, of electronic gadgets and time-saving machinery, we still have much the same body as our ancestors, the Stone Age man. It took millions of years of evolution for the human body to become adapted for primitive survival – for running, jumping, fighting, lifting, dragging, climbing – in order to hunt, trap and gather food. It simply hasn't had time to adapt to our mollycoddled way of life. Your body was designed for vigorous daily activity, and it misses it. For the body to function correctly, constant activity of all parts is essential.

To be perfectly fit for life, there are many aspects of our daily routine which must be taken into consideration, not simply exercise, but diet, digestion, rest, and freedom from abuse are important too. All the fluids of our body, the blood and lymph, also need to be kept in constant circulation, and this is why exercise is so vital. We tend to think that by doing exercises only our limbs and muscles will benefit, and forget that at the same time the heart, kidneys, glands, skin, and other organs of the body will all be strengthened, and so function more efficiently.

So, what is fitness, and how do we know if we are really fit? True fitness is more than simply being able to cope with the stresses and strains of everyday life. It consists of three important ingredients – stamina, suppleness, and strength – known as the S-Factors:

Stamina: This is staying power, endurance, the ability to keep going without gasping for breath. For stamina you need a well-developed circulation in the heart and lungs, so that plenty of vital oxygen is pumped to your working muscles. With stamina you have a slower and much more powerful heartbeat. You can cope more easily with prolonged or heavy exertion, and you'll be less likely to suffer from killer heart disease.

Suppleness: This means being flexible and developing a maximum range of body movements without spraining ligaments and pulling muscles and tendons. The more mobile and supple you are, the less likely you'll suffer aches and pains brought on by stiffness.

Strength: This is extra muscle-power in reserve for those often unexpected heavier jobs. Lifting and shifting need strong shoulder, trunk and thigh muscles. Toned-up tummy muscles also help to take the strain . . . and keep your waistline trim.

At school we learnt the three R's, and now it is necessary to learn the three S's. Exercise is obviously essential, but don't sit back in your chair and groan that you're too old, you haven't got time, or you're quite happy as you are: here are some very good reasons why you should start exercising today:

1   To protect your heart: Exercise will stimulate your body's own natural maintenance and repair system. Your bones, joints and muscles, and especially your heart, will actually stay younger if you keep them busy. Research has shown that people who take enough regular vigorous exercise can cut their risk of suffering a heart attack.

2   To stay slim and improve your physical appearance: Exercise is an important part of weight control, and will help you stay slim. It uses up energy, which comes from the calories you eat. The number of calories you burn up depends both on how rigorous the exercise is, and how long you keep it up. For example, an hour's walking uses about the same number of calories as half-an-hour's hard swimming. But apart from that, some experts believe that regular exercise may help you slim even while you sleep, by

speeding up the overall rate at which your body burns up calories.

3 Coping with stress: Gentle rhythmic exercise – like swimming, cycling or jogging – is a superb way of releasing tension caused by the stress of everyday life. Mind and body relax into the rhythm, and stress is eased away. Also, the feeling of tiredness – not exhaustion – brought on by physical effort may help to promote deep and refreshing sleep.

To remain physically and mentally active throughout our lives, it is important to remain healthy and fit. The average life span today is around seventy-seven years of age, many killer diseases can now be cured, or at least controlled, so it is within our power to make the very best of ourselves and not only look good, but feel good, and be able to do exactly what we want to do. To achieve total fitness doesn't mean you have to be a fanatic and take things too seriously, but it does mean being sensible about things and looking after your body.

Always remember when exercising to start slowly, and never rush into them or strain yourself, as this will obviously do far more harm than good. Even top athletes, if they have had a short break from their sport, begin their training slowly and work their way up, although they know they are capable of doing more, and this is how you must be too. I am quite active and always run up stairs rather than use a lift, but I'm not fit in the sense that I could get in the ring and start boxing again. That would mean months of hard training, starting off gradually and working my way up.

Well, how fit do *you* feel? The most important tests of fitness are those that measure stamina and involve rhythmic movement of large groups of muscles for sustained periods. But people differ in the amount of physical effort they need to make to achieve a reasonable level of fitness. It depends upon your general state of health

4

too. It would be very stupid to rush into vigorous exercise that may aggravate a medical condition. And, of course, it depends on how fit you already are. Great care must be taken before starting to exercise, and although most people, even the elderly, will not need a medical check-up, it is advisable to consult a doctor if:

1 You suffer from high blood pressure or heart disease.
2 You have chest trouble, like asthma or bronchitis.
3 You're troubled with joint pains, such as back aches or arthritis.
4 You're recovering from an illness or operation.

Never exercise after a meal as this puts an extra strain upon your heart and digestion. You will find that champion athletes always exercise on an empty stomach. Many people believe exercise is best done in the morning too, as this will stimulate the metabolism and make you feel great for the rest of the day. When I was boxing I used to start training at 4 o'clock in the morning, exercise for a couple of hours and be sweated out and showered and back in bed by six. I could then have two or three hours sleep until 9 o'clock when I would breakfast, and be ready for the day ahead.

To test just how fit you are, here are four simple tests. The first one you should find quite easy. Tests 2 and 3 are a little more demanding, and Test 4 should not be attempted unless you are sure that you are reasonably fit already. If not, you may feel that you will need a few weeks of gentle exercise first to get you back into shape.

Do remember to start gently and build up gradually. There are no prizes for winning, this isn't a contest, it's just a simple test to see how fit you really are.

Test 1

Try walking up and down a flight of stairs (about fifteen steps) *three* times fairly briskly. You should be able to hold an ordinary conversation without being at all out of breath.

Test 2

Run on the spot. Lifting your feet at least six inches (15cm) off the floor. Keep going until you feel a bit short of breath or tired, then stop. Don't force yourself. If you are over fifty you should be able to manage two minutes quite comfortably. Younger people should find three minutes quite easy.

Test 3

Using either the second step of the stairs or a firm bench or strong chair, step up and down briskly, alternating your leading foot. Stop as soon as you feel a bit puffed or tired. Again, don't force yourself to keep going. If you're over fifty and reasonably fit you should be able to hold a conversation without being too short of breath after two minutes of stepping. A fit under-fifty-year-old should still be able to manage this after three minutes.

Test 4

Don't try this until you can do Test 3 comfortably. Jog gently and easily for one mile (you can measure it using a car milometer). The time given to cover the distance depends upon your age:

> Under 45 – ten minutes for men, twelve for women.
> Over 45 – add a minute for every five years.

Throughout the test, and immediately afterwards, you should be able to hold an ordinary conversation without being too out of breath.

This is only a general guide, but people in the lowest group must exercise very gradually (five minutes per day), and slowly increase over the months to ten or fifteen minutes a day as the heartrate improves.

What is Exercise?

Exercise is the name we give to any muscular activity which will cause a change in bodily functions, especially those of the heart and lungs. The extent of these changes depends upon the type and severity of the exercise and the fitness of the individual.

'High Resistance exercise' is physical activity involving sustained muscle contractions as in weight-lifting or 'press-ups'. Such exercise can be dangerous for people with heart disease or high blood pressure because of the resulting strain on the heart.

'Dynamic exercise' is physical activity in which muscles contract or shorten in a rhythmic manner, such as when running, jogging, walking and swimming. Whichever activity you choose it is essential to do it regularly, so it must be something you enjoy!

As a simple rule, exercise should be enough to cause very mild breathlessness. A bout of exercise should last three to five minutes to give an appreciable training effect on the functions of the heart and lungs. Bouts should be repeated at five minute intervals in half-hour sessions at least twice a week.

Always select varied physical activities which you can enjoy without discomfort and in which you can progressively increase your effort. You can take a considerable amount of exercise unobtrusively by walking or cycling to work, avoiding escalators and lifts in favour of walking up stairs. If you are under thirty-five years of age you can begin exercising straight away, although gradually at first. If you are over thirty-five and have not exercised since you left school, then start gradually, but if you are worried about exercise symptoms consult your doctor.

Remember that it is continued and continuous effort that counts in keeping fit, not rushing into an hour's exercise in one day and then leaving it for a month – that will do far more harm than good. If you are really out of condition then take things very easy and work up very slowly to a regular session each day.

Whatever your condition, choose your exercises carefully. There are some here for everyone, whether you are a jet-setting businessman or a housebound housewife, and don't forget about relaxation too. In a world of stress and tension it is just as important to your health to learn how to relax after your exercises.

Don't forget that fitness should be fun too! Don't feel that you are adding on the years, but that you are making yourself really fit for life.

Chapter Two

Building Up a Fitness Routine

The most important thing about getting fit is starting NOW. It is no good thinking 'Oh, I'll be fit one day'. While you are busy deciding what you can do and when you can do it, try going for a walk. Then go for another . . . and another . . . and before you even realise it you will be on your way!

While walking don't dawdle, but walk confidently and swing your body loosely in its natural rhythm. Brisk walking, especially up hill, is a marvellous exercise for the heart and lungs. Your stamina can soon be built up by a few brisk walks a day, and if you are over forty then this is a particularly safe exercise and is a good way to get back into shape. If you have got a dog, then take him with you for he'll appreciate the exercise too.

You can soon make walking a part of your daily routine. If you live within walking distance from work, then why bother to wait in the bus queue, when with a little bit of effort you could walk almost as quickly. If it is too far to walk *all* the way to work, then try walking part of the way and walk to the next bus stop. It will save you money too.

Take a walk at lunchtime too, even if it is just round a park or the nearest shops. If you can walk up stairs rather than take a lift, then do. Just five minutes a day of climbing stairs can help to keep your heart and lungs in trim.

At weekends, or when you have more time to spare, go for longer walks, preferably up hills. Or if you haven't any hills nearby, go to your nearest golf course and play a round. Golf is now my first love so, in my spare time, I like to be on the golf course where there is plenty of fresh air, and I get plenty of exercise in pursuit of that little white ball! It's possible to walk a couple of miles in each round without even noticing it.

If you do not want to brave the elements to exercise, then you can keep yourself perfectly fit with very simple activities, such as running on the spot, skipping, or even dancing to your favourite records on the radio. Try five or ten minutes of disco style dancing every day, but make sure the neighbours aren't watching!

By doing vigorous exercise, even as little as thirty minutes three days a week, we can build up the efficiency of our heart and strengthen our muscles and improve the circulation. Many experts believe that regular exercise protects us from coronary heart disease by preventing blockage of the blood vessels which serve the heart. Few people realise that the heart is a special kind of muscle and can be increased in size, strength and efficiency. Despite popular belief, doctors confirm that heart weakness comes not from overworking the heart, but from abuses such as drinking, smoking, and gluttony. A fatty heart, is what must be avoided at all costs. Exercise will make the heart beat faster and, therefore, strengthen it. With a strong heart you will be fit to tackle anything.

Once you have decided how fit you are, or how fit you are not, you may feel that you would like to embark on a regular exercise routine to keep yourself in trim. Some people prefer to follow a set schedule of exercises on which they can spend a few minutes each day. But if you feel you cannot face a daily exercise discipline then try every other day, which is roughly three times a week, and you'll soon feel the benefit.

So, now you're ready to begin. Do remember not to work too hard too soon. Muscles are meant to be elastic, but if you're out of condition they won't be, so work up your exercise routine gradually. A little every day is much better than a violent burst of activity every now and again.

Start by doing each exercise two or three times, and increase the number daily. Even if you feel you can do more, don't. You'll know if you are overdoing things

10

because you will feel very stiff the next day. So ease yourself in gradually, that is the secret.

Here is a simple daily routine that will increase your mobility and strength, and exercise your heart and lungs. It will tone up your muscles, deepen your breathing, improve circulation and posture. It will not only make you feel good, but look good too.

Daily Exercise Routine

Exercise 1: Arm Swinging. Begin with your legs wide apart and your arms hanging loosely by your side. Raise both your arms forwards, upwards, backwards and downwards, in a circular motion, brushing your ears with your arms as you go past. A very good exercise for your arm muscles and shoulders, and will help improve posture.

Exercise 2: Side bends. Again, stand with your legs apart. Place your hands on your hips. Now bend first to the left and then to the right.

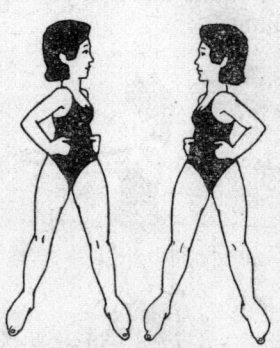

Exercise 3: Trunk, knee and hip bends. Stand approximately eighteen inches behind the back of a chair, with your hands resting very lightly on the back. Raise your left knee and bring your forehead down to meet it so that they actually touch, if possible. Do not rush; this must be a long, strong

movement. When you are used to the action, you can dispense with the chair and work from a standing position. Try this five to eight times to begin with and gradually increase the number each day.

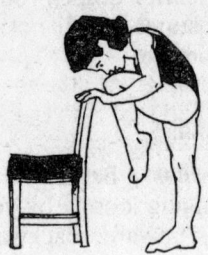

Exercise 4: Head, arms and trunk rotation. Stand with your feet astride and both your arms straight out in front of you at shoulder level. Turn your head, arms and shoulders around to the left as far as you can go, bending the right arm across your chest. Then repeat, this time turning towards the right. Make sure that you keep your hips and legs still throughout.

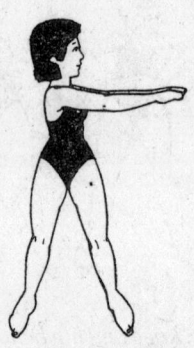

Exercise 5: Alternate ankle reach. Stand with both feet wide apart, and both palms on the front of the upper left thigh. Relax the trunk forward as you slide both hands down the

front of your leg towards your foot, grasp your ankle for a count of five and return to the upright position. Then do the same with the right leg. If you suffer from even very mild back trouble only put your hands as far as your knees.

Exercise 6: Wall press-ups. Stand with your hands on a wall at shoulder height, approximately twelve inches apart. Make sure that your arms are straight out in front of you. Stand on your toes and lean forward, bending your arms, until your chin and chest touch the wall. Return to your original position by straightening your arms. Do this eight to ten times at first and gradually increase daily until you are doing twenty five to thirty.

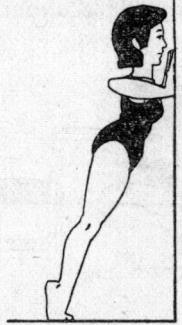

Exercise 7: Abdominal exercise. This will help flatten your tummy muscles. Sit on the front part of a chair, legs

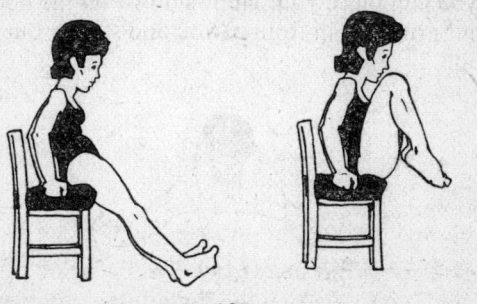

13

straight, heels on the floor. Lean back and grip the sides of the seat for support. Bend the knees and bring the fronts of the thighs up to squeeze gently against the body. (You can also do the same exercise with the legs held straight – if you're Olga Korbut!)

Exercise 8: Leg exercise. Stand eighteen inches behind a chair with your hands on the back. Keeping your spine perfectly straight, lower the body into a squat, keeping the feet flat on the floor. (If you find this difficult it will help to have a half or one inch block under your heels.) Straighten both legs and come up on the toes, then return to the squat position. As you become more experienced you can dispense with the chair and place your hands on your hips.

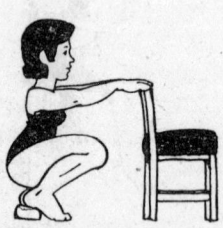

Exercise 9: Spinal stretch. Sit on the floor with your legs as wide apart as they will go. Begin by leaning forward, and see if you can place your elbows down on the floor. Then put your arms out in front of you and stretch out as far as you can.

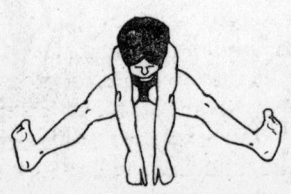

Exercise 10: Running on the spot. At the end of your session stand with your arms loosely by your side and run gently on the spot. Do not raise your knees very high, but aim to raise them higher as you progress. Start very gradually, say for about thirty seconds, and build it up daily.

With most fitness routines the incentive to persist is very weak and we give up before any noticeable improvement can be seen. This routine, however, is designed to exercise each part of the body in turn and it should not be long before you begin to notice the difference. If you set aside a particular time each day for exercise, and stick to that time each day, you will soon find that it naturally becomes part of your normal routine. Also you will not have to spend hours exercising daily; these exercises take just a few minutes to do, and even three times a week will help.

If you couple these exercises with a little conscientious effort in your daily life – such as walking whenever possible – you will certainly feel the difference. Other factors must also be taken into consideration too, such as food and sleep, and you will find these matters dealt with later in the book.

Don't take any notice of the old maxim that, if an exercise hurts, it is doing you good; that is not true. Always underestimate your capabilities and do a little less than you think you can. You will find that you progress much more quickly than rushing into vigorous exercise and finding yourself as stiff as a board for the next couple of days. Listen to your body, it is the best judge of what you can do, and don't strain it because it is the only one you've got!

You will discover that with regular exercise you will sleep much better too, and exercise and rest go hand in hand to make you fit. You may find that in your daily routine the only time you have available for exercise is at night. OK, not to worry. Do your exercise routine, and follow it with a nice relaxing bath, and you will find that your sleep will be much more sound.

Before starting your exercises, be sure to have a general

limbering up session. This is necessary, not only for people in poor condition, but for accomplished athletes too. In the next section you will find a series of limbering up exercises that will be useful. Warming up in this way prepares your body for exercise and it aids the circulation and nervous response. If you simply rush into exercise your body will be unprepared and this could put a strain on the heart and lungs, whereas if you warm up and are prepared you will find the exercises that much easier.

Remember that your muscles are what we call 'antagonistic' – this means that they work opposite each other so that when one contracts the other relaxes, so be sure to make all parts of the body stretch to their fullest, not just one side of the body, or one leg. The more a muscle is contracted the more it will relax afterwards, and the more you will gain from the exercises.

Breathing

Finally, whilst exercising, do pay particular attention to your breathing. On average we tend to use less than fifty per cent of our full lung capacity, which is really like inflation – you've got £1 but you only get 50p in value out of it! If you want to use every penny of your money, which most of us do, why not make full use of your lungs and feel better too.

It is usually when we do something strenuous and gasp for breath that we become conscious of our lungs.

Try placing your hands on your chest and make yourself fully aware of *how* you actually breathe. The best way is to use the diaphragm. If you don't know where that is, place the palms of your hands just below your rib cage with the finger tips lightly touching and as you breathe in, your finger tips will be pulled apart. Actors who have to throw their voice to the back of a theatre learn to breathe with their diaphragm because this makes the most of their lung capacity. Obviously it is a difficult matter to change the *way* in which you breathe because you've been doing it since you were born. But do be conscious of your breathing and as it becomes faster during exercise try and control it by using your diaphragm. You will find this will not only aid your oxygen intake, but it will strengthen and tighten your stomach muscles. It will also help your posture as you will find that with a good, straight back you will be able to breathe much more deeply and efficiently.

Here is a breathing exercise which will encourage you to make complete use of your lungs:

Correct breathing. Breathe out completely so that your lungs are as empty as you can get them, then slowly inhale through the nose at a slow count of five. Just let your abdomen swell. Then breathe in for another count of five, this time letting your rib cage expand. Place your hands on your rib cage throughout this exercise so that you can feel exactly what is happening. Exhale very slowly to a count of ten through your mouth, feeling how the rib cage shrinks and your abdomen (diaphragm) tightens. The diaphragm tightens during INspiration and relaxes during EXpiration.

If you do this ten times daily, you will find it not only makes you totally aware of how you breathe, but it will also relax your muscles and give you more energy. If you get very tense, or nervous, (perhaps you are worried about a driving test or a visit to the dentist), try this exercise and it will make you feel calm and much relaxed. But be warned: don't keep on doing it or you'll pass out!

With just a little practice you will soon find that you are breathing correctly without even thinking about it.

Chapter Three

Limbering Up and Exercises At Home

Before doing any exercise it is important that you have
limbered up and that your muscles are ready for action.
Just like you, they need coaxing gently and if they have
been inactive for some time then you don't want to shock
them too much by plunging straight into vigorous exercise.
Otherwise they might just let you know how they feel by
giving you a sharp pain in protest the next day!

Spend two or three minutes before each session
limbering up. This not only helps to keep your joints
flexible, but also tones up all your major muscle groups by
stretching them a little. Rather like a cat stretching itself
before springing into action. You will also find that a good
stretch *after* your exercises will make you feel really fit and
able to cope with anything.

Here are five simple movements to do in an easy and
unhurried way, gently stretching each action without
forcing it. Repeat each movement ten times, breathing
normally all the time.

Exercise 1: Head rolling. Stand with your feet apart, hands
on hips, and spine straight. Tip your head back and look up
at the ceiling. Very slowly roll your head round to the right
in a circular movement until you are looking at the floor.
Now roll it round to the left until you are looking at the
floor on the other side and back again so that you are
looking at the ceiling once more. Your head will then have
done a complete circle. Repeat in the opposite direction.
This really is a very enjoyable exercise and has a massaging
effect on your neck and shoulders, although it is perhaps
inadvisable for the elderly. You should check with your
doctor first.

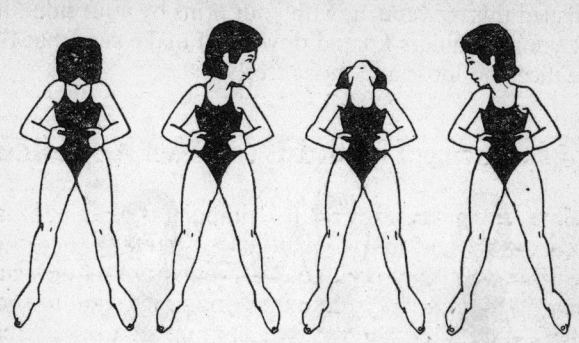

Exercise 2: Side bending. With feet still apart and hands on your sides, lean first to the right, and then to the left, sliding the hand down the side of the leg. This will stretch your spine and make it more supple. Keep your feet firmly on the floor while doing this – don't cheat!

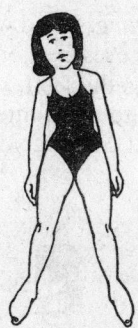

Exercise 3: Arm swinging. Still standing with your feet apart, push both arms out in front of you, finger tips touching, raise them above your head and then out to your side, pushing each arm backward at the same time. Then, with your arms out in front of you move them up above your head, behind you, and forward again in a circular motion. Repeat in the opposite direction. You will feel this making your shoulder blades very supple. When you have

finished this movement, with your arms by your sides, just lift your shoulders up and down and make sure that they are nice and loose and move freely.

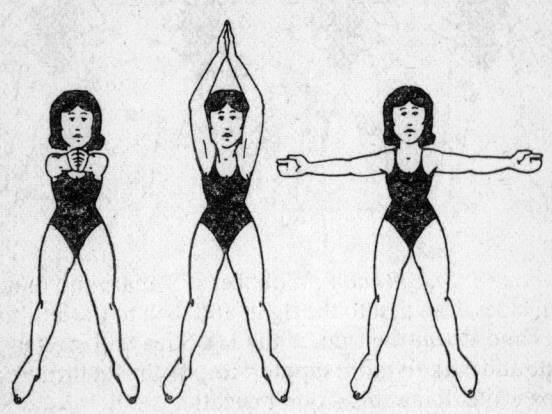

Exercise 4: Trunk twisting. Stand with feet apart and arms out in front. With your eyes fixed on your right hand, swing your right arm round to the right, keeping it straight, as far as it will go. Return it to the front and repeat with the left arm. You will feel that twisting your spine makes it more flexible.

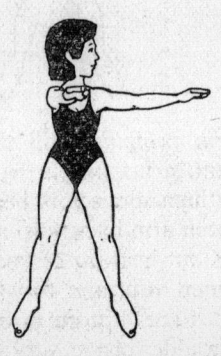

Exercise 5: Hip flexing. Stand with your feet together. Bring one knee up to your chest, pulling it with your hands if necessary. Then bow your head and touch your knee with your forehead. Repeat with the other knee.

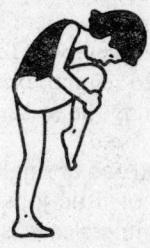

Exercise 6: Back arching. Stand with your legs apart and knees slightly bent. Try and keep your hips in the same position, but bend forward as far as you can. Then straighten up and arch backwards, again try not to move your hips. You will now have flexed your spine in every direction.

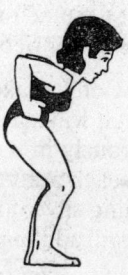

You should now be warmed up and ready for action. Do these limbering up exercises before any vigorous activity, whether it is a session of fitness exercises or any of your favourite sports or athletics that you may be participating in. This will mean that your muscles will not be cold and your heart and lungs will be in full swing and ready to tackle anything.

Exercises at Home

Many people feel that they simply cannot face a regular exercise routine, or know deep down that however good their intentions may be, they will give up after a short time. If you fall into that category, there's no need to give up the idea of exercise completely. Obviously it would be beneficial for you to do regular exercises, but if you really can't, then try combining the tasks you perform every day in the home with exercise.

Whether you are married or single, male or female, there are always hundreds of little jobs in the home that can easily be turned into fitness exercises, and the housework can become more fun than you ever thought possible!

Here are just a few of the chores that can make you fit; you will probably be able to think of a lot more . . .

Dusting. Try dusting with a feather duster, one that is not too long, and reach up and dust all the high points in your house: the top shelves that you usually ignore, the tops of wardrobes which will really cause you to stretch, tops of doors, and don't forget to stand on tip-toe and reach right into the corners in case of cobwebs.

Polishing. This will not only make all your furniture and mirrors really shine but it will make your arm muscles firm and strong. Rub vigorously in a circular movement, and use both hands so that each arm receives the same amount of exercise. Try polishing silver and cutlery too. This will take a lot of effort, but will add sparkle to your home and to your physique.

Scrubbing. Very few people actually scrub floors today. I can remember my grandmothers scrubbing steps and kitchen floors. My gran on my mother's side lived until she was 84 and my father's mother lived until she was 87, so it obviously didn't do them any harm! So if you've got a dirty front door step, then give it a good scrub once in a while, and getting down on your hands and knees to clean the kitchen floor can exercise your spine, legs, arms and neck. Dispose of the mop and squeegee! When it is dry try giving it a good polish too, but kneel on a cushion to save unnecessary pain to your knees.

Washing up. To celebrate that you have finished washing-up do a few exercises against the sink top! Especially the leg exercise (Exercise 8) in the previous chapter. Concentrate on how you put the dishes away – if they are in low cupboards then bend the knees, not the back, and go down in a squat position, keeping the spine straight. Where possible, stretch to put things in high cupboards.

Hanging out washing. In this day of tumbledriers few people actually hang out washing, but if you do have a washing line then take advantage of it on a warm summer's day to get some exercise. Make sure that it is as high as it will go so that you really have to stretch to put your washing on it.

Making beds. Of all the household jobs, making a bed is always considered to be one of the most strenuous, and can certainly make even a fit person breathless. If possible get someone to help you, husbands and wives can exercise together. Always face the bed squarely, keeping the back stiff where possible. Practice some knee bends too while you are tucking the sheets in.

Cleaning windows. A combination exercise that involves stretching. Try not to stand on a chair or steps until you have really cleaned and stretched as high as you possibly can. As with polishing this will also strengthen the arms and wrists if you use a circular movement. For ladies it is a good exercise for firming the bust.

Skirting boards. Get down on your knees again to dust your skirting boards. Kneel about two feet away from the wall and lean forward to dust the skirting board, stretching as far as you can to the left and right before moving your position.

Cooking. You can easily devise your own exercises whilst cooking, depending upon what it is you are doing: whether you are tenderising steak with a mallet, using a hand beater whilst making a cake, rolling pastry, stirring, chopping, or peeling, all involve particular muscular movement, so use it to its best advantage.

So, you see that simple everyday housework can be turned into fitness exercises. Obviously there will be no instant, startling differences, but every little helps and anything is better than nothing, and will certainly help you in your battle to keep fit.

Exercising in the Garden

If you have a garden you will know that there are always plenty of jobs to be done all the year round, and I expect that at some time or another, after a couple of hours gardening, you have been as stiff as a poker for a week! If, however, you work properly then gardening can be a very good method of toning up the muscles and if you don't overdo things there is no reason at all why you should suffer.

The major reason why people are stiff and aching after gardening is because they spend too long at one particular job. Don't spend all afternoon digging, because your back and arms will suffer. Instead do some digging, then some pruning, some weeding, a little more digging, and so on. You'll find that the work gets done just as quickly, and a change is as good as a rest, so you won't get bored with one job.

Digging. A marvellous exercise for the legs, arms, and spine, but be careful not to stoop whilst digging. Keep the spine as straight as possible, and every now and again flex the spine forward and back in an arch, like a cat, and this will keep the spine very supple.

24

Hoeing. As with digging, look after your back. Any activity such as hoeing or raking can be a relaxing exercise if done rhythmically, so swing and bend your knees whilst you work. This will keep your joints mobile.

Weeding. This usually causes stiff backs and sore knees, so don't stay in one position too long. Make sure that you have something comfortable to kneel on, and after kneeling for a time, try squatting. Keep your spine as straight as possible and move from side to side as you work.

Hedge trimming. Use hand shears rather then electric trimmers and you will find that the action required will strengthen your arms and tone up your shoulders and chest. Again, don't spend too long at it, and be sure to have a really good stretch afterwards to relax all the muscles. Remember about them being 'antagonistic'? In a job such as this you tend to have many of the same muscles contracted, so a good stretch is required to stop them getting stiff.

Fruit picking. If you are lucky enough to have fruit trees, then don't wait for the fruit to fall and damage your back by bending down to pick it up! When it is ripe and ready for picking, stand on the ground, on tip-toe if necessary, and stretch up high and pick as much as you can, having a really good stretch. If any fruit is on the ground, then pick it up by bending the knees and going down to it that way.

Planting. If you are planting bulbs or small plants, don't stoop. Get right down to it and put down something comfortable to kneel on, or try sitting with your legs as far apart as possible and lean forward, keeping your spine perfectly straight. Don't worry what the neighbours think! You'll soon be fit enough to leap over the fence and give them some of your garden produce.

Cutting the grass. If you have a conventional hand mower, so much the better. This will require some effort to push and so strengthen your arm and leg muscles. Even if it is a motor-mower, keep your back perfectly straight as you go around and don't stoop over it. If it is a motor-mower then you can make good use of its pulling action to strengthen your arms by letting it pull away from you.

Any gardening activities should be used to their best advantage and if you check your movements and posture wisely, then good use can be made of the work, not only in making your garden productive, but in keeping you in peak condition. As well as being exercised you will also be breathing in plenty of fresh air, and sometimes you will feel the benefit of the sun's rays too.

If it does happen to be very sunny then take special precautions against over exposure to sunlight. This can have a drying effect on the skin, so, if you have a dry skin anyway, put on a protective cream or sun oil. Wear a hat if possible, and if it happens to be very hot then do not spend too many hours in the garden at a time. It is very easy to burn the skin without realising it, and sunburn can be very painful. To replace any water lost through perspiration, in a normal day we lose about half a pint of sweat and with exercise this can be more, drink plenty of fluid.

A few hours in the garden can make you feel invigorated and full of energy, and will burn up those excess calories too.

Armchair Exercises

If you do not have a garden, have little housework to do, or are just too lazy to get out of a chair, don't worry! You can exercise too. While you're watching TV you might as well keep fit at the same time, especially if the programme is boring. Also if you happen to be confined to bed, then some of these exercises might be useful to you too.

Exercise 1: Toe stretch. Sit with your legs straight out in front of you and try and separate all your toes, spreading them wide apart. This isn't as easy as it sounds and will require a great deal of concentration. Once you have mastered that, wiggle your toes *separately*, starting with the big toe and keeping the others still, then the next toe, and so on. You will find that this requires even greater concentration, so try keeping your other foot perfectly still and wiggle only one toe out of ten at a time!

Exercise 2: Foot strengthener. Again with your legs stretched out in front of you, toes together, point your feet downwards as far as they will go (as if someone had laid a heavy book on your feet). Then point them upwards towards your knees as though you were pushing your heels firmly down. You will feel a strong pull at the backs of your legs when you do this. Finally, turn the soles of your feet inwards and see if you can press them together, heel against heel, big toe against big toe, and so on.

Exercise 3: Ankle strengthener. Lift your feet six inches off the ground, making sure your legs are straight, and gently rotate your ankle in a clockwise direction five times. Then repeat in an anti-clockwise direction. Finally rotate your left leg in an anti-clockwise direction and your right leg in a clockwise direction. You will find that this not only strengthens your ankles but helps the blood circulation in your legs too. As an exercise this is especially valuable for those confined to bed.

Exercise 4: Limb strengthener. Lift your legs straight out in front of you very slowly, as high as you can so that you feel a slight pull in the stomach muscles. Now open and close your legs ten times in a scissor-like action. Then rotate your legs, as you did with the ankles but this time the whole leg, in a circular motion.

Now, placing your legs back on to the floor, put your legs very close together, knees touching, and slowly lift them as high as you can.

Similar exercises can be done with the arms, try rotating

27

them too, especially the wrists, and the fingers can be strengthened by doing the toe exercises.

Exercise 5: Trunk firmer. In your sitting position try squeezing the buttocks together as firmly as you can, hold for one minute and then relax. This will help firm the muscles. Then try squeezing your stomach muscles in, pull as tight as you can so that your stomach is flat and hold for a minute. Breathe in as you do so and let the air out very slowly, but don't let your tummy muscles relax as you breathe out. Again this will firm up your stomach. These exercises can be done anywhere, on a train, plane, or bus, because no-one will see what you are doing and, who knows, they might be squeezing their buttocks together too!

While sitting, whether it is watching TV or on a bus, try and keep your spine straight. Sit for a time on the edge of your seat, and be sure not to slouch. This will make the back firm and improve your posture. Rotate your shoulders in a clockwise direction so that they are being pulled back.

Exercise 6: Head and neck contractions. Clasp your fingers together, put your hands behind your head and press your head back as hard as you can and hold for a count of ten. Relax for ten and repeat. This will help tone the neck muscles.

Now, give your neck muscles a good stretch by leaning your head back as far as it will possibly go, and slowly bring it forward as far as it will go, so that your chin is on your chest. Aim to get your nose on your chest – it is physically impossible to do, but it will give you the right movement.

Bring your head to an upright position. Lay it slowly on one side so that your right ear touches your right shoulder. Slowly move it back to upright and across to the left.

To complete the neck exercises, with your head facing front, turn and look over your right shoulder as far as you can, keeping your body facing forward. Slowly turn your head back to the front and round so that you look over your left shoulder.

If you are alone in the room, you can do a few facial exercises! I say if you're on your own, because anyone else in the room might think you are being very rude!

Start by opening your mouth as wide as it will go and stick your tongue right out, further than you've ever put it out before. You will really feel the stretch. Put your tongue back in your mouth. Now put your mouth into a really wide grin and hold for a count of five. Then purse your lips forward as though you were going to give someone a big kiss and hold that for a count of five. Alternate the two movements quickly, going from a grin to a kiss, twelve times.

Finally, exercise your facial muscles by first screwing your face up as tightly as you can, wrinkle your nose, screw up your eyes, your mouth, and then slowly let it relax. Now stretch your face out by raising your eyebrows, opening your eyes wide, and opening your mouth. This will keep your face supple and tone up the muscles.

Physical Exercises

For those of you who don't want to take the easy way out, and would prefer some really practical physical exercises to keep the body in shape, then this section is for you. Here are some random exercises for all parts of the body, and from these you can pick out the ones most appropriate to your own condition (perhaps you have bad posture, for example), and from these make up your own daily exercise routine. As with all exercises, don't rush into them or do too many to start with, and be sure to do some limbering up first before you embark on your routine.

Exercises for the abdomen. The abdomen is an area of the body that does not get exercised in our normal daily life, unlike our arms and legs, and so it is important to do specific exercises to strengthen this area of the body.

a: Lie down on the floor with your arms by your side and your legs stretched out in front of you. Keeping your head and back on the floor, slowly raise your legs about one foot off the floor. Hold for a count of five, and slowly lower them again. The next day raise them nine inches off the floor, then six, until after about a week you are able to raise your legs only three inches off the floor and hold them there for a count of five – or even ten.

b: Do the previous exercise in reverse. So this time you must keep your feet, legs, and buttocks firmly on the floor, and very slowly raise your head and trunk, come right forward and touch your toes. The secret is going back *slowly*. You will find that this also strengthens your back. As with the last exercise, be sure not to do too many until you become supple and mobile again.

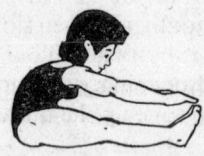

c: Lie on your back and raise your legs in the air, supporting your hips with your hands, and try and do a shoulder stand by raising your legs vertically in the air. Once you have become experienced at shoulder stands, slowly bring your legs over and try and touch the floor with your toes. This will give you a good spinal stretch too.

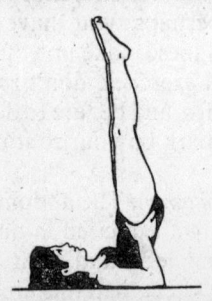

d: Whilst in a shoulder stand pretend that you are riding a bicycle and 'pedal' with your legs for a count of fifty. You will feel the pull on your abdomen, and your legs will be strengthened too.

e: Lying flat on your back, lift your knees up to your chest and twist them to the right so that they touch the floor, and then to the left. Throughout this exercise, keep your head and shoulders firmly on the floor.

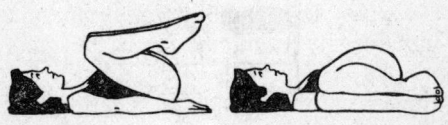

Exercises for posture:

a: Stand upright with your spine as straight as possible, place your arms behind your back so that your hands are level with your buttocks and clasp your fingers together. Keeping your arms perfectly straight lift your hands into the air so that your shoulder blades touch. You will feel a good stretch in the shoulders and the back of your neck.

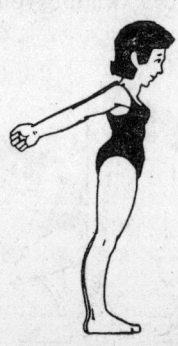

31

b: Sit on a chair, with your spine straight, clasp your hands behind your head and try and force your elbows out and back so that they are as wide apart as possible.

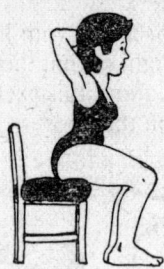

c: Lie face downwards on the floor, and raising just your head and shoulders from the floor, try and get your head back as far as you can so that you are looking at the ceiling.

d: Stand upright with your hands on your hips and keeping your lower half perfectly straight, turn the top half of your body as far as you can to the right, and then the same to the left. This will exercise muscles at the side of your spine which are not normally used.

e: Stand with your back against a wall, your feet firmly together, and your heels about twelve inches from the wall. Keeping the small of your back flat against the wall bend down and touch your toes, bending your knees at the same time.

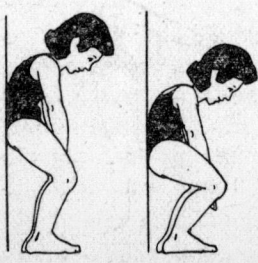

f: Lying face downwards on the floor, reach behind you and grasp your ankles, pull them off the floor, raising your head and chest at the same time so that your body is supported by your abdomen.

Exercises for limbs:

a: To make your leg muscles really firm, stand at right angles to a wall and press on to it with your left hand. Now swing your right leg as far forward as you can, and then back as far as it will go. Keep it swinging, like a pendulum. Then repeat with the other side. Make sure that you have plenty of room for this and that you're not going to damage yourself by kicking into furniture!

b: Standing perfectly straight, with your feet eighteen inches apart and arms hanging loosely by your side, raise yourself up onto your toes and bending the knees, go down into a squatting position so that you are actually sitting on your heels. Be sure that the spine is kept erect throughout.

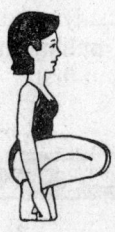

c: An exercise that will involve your arms as well as your legs is to stand with your feet flat on the floor, back straight, arms by your side. Swing your arms up in the air, over your head and at the same time come up on your toes like a ballet dancer. As you bring your arms down, bring your heels down too. Practice this swinging movement fifteen to twenty times to begin with. It's a good limbering up exercise too.

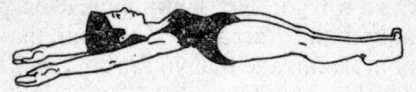

d: Lie on the floor on your right side with your right arm
straight out above your head and support yourself with
your left hand. Lift your legs a couple of inches off the floor,
from the hips, and try a pedalling movement, as if you were
riding a bicycle. Then turn over and try it on your left side.
You will find this especially good for your thighs and hips,
and may find a bit of pulling in your pelvic muscles, so
don't be too strenuous at first.

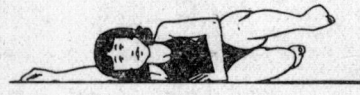

e: Sit on the floor with your legs about eighteen inches
apart. Keeping your back straight, reach forward and
grasp your left ankle with both hands and pull your left leg
up as high as it will go. Keep the leg perfectly straight, and
remember to keep your right leg on the floor throughout.
You will feel a real pull on your thighs and ham-strings.
Don't worry if you cannot get the leg very high to start
with, you will find that each time you exercise you will be
able to go just that little bit further until you can bring your
ankle up to touch your nose. Now repeat with the other leg.

f: Press-ups are excellent for your arm muscles. Lie face down on the floor with your palms flat. Now push yourself up by straightening your arms and let the arms support the weight of your body. Lower yourself down very slowly, don't just collapse on the floor, and when you get within an inch of the floor, hold the position for a moment and feel the pull in your arms.

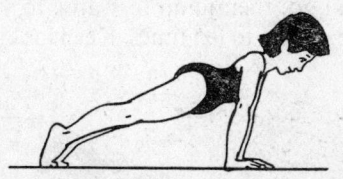

g: Lie down in a position as if you were going to do press-ups, and keeping the palms of your hands firmly on the floor, get up and walk towards them. Go as far as you can, keeping the legs straight and your heels on the floor.

h: Although one of the simplest exercises of all, there is nothing to beat running on the spot for strengthening your legs and your arms. Try running slowly to begin with and increase it as you get fitter. Swing your arms in a natural rhythmical running movement too, so that they get the full benefit of the exercise.

General fitness exercises.

a: Stand with the spine straight and your feet slightly apart. Place the palms of your hands on your chest so that your elbows are both pointing outwards. Move your elbows in a circular movement in a clockwise direction ten times and then anti-clockwise. Try and make as big a circle as you can.

b: Jump into the air opening your legs as far as they will go and raising your arms as you jump. Land with your feet together, and your arms by your side. Once you get the basic rhythm you can do fifteen to twenty of these. Very good for the heart and lungs. (If you are a newcomer to this exercise it can cause thigh stiffness, so introduce yourself to it gradually.)

c: Bend down in a crouching position with your hands in front of you on the floor. Keeping your hands in the same position, jump backwards, putting your feet as far behind you as they will go, then jump forwards to your original position. Do this eight to ten times. Keep looking ahead all the time.

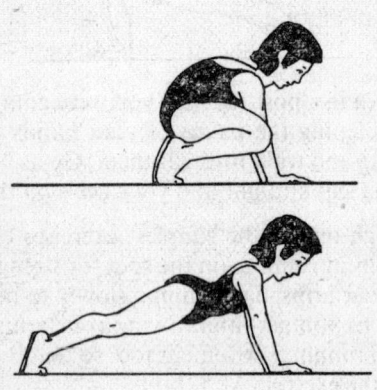

d: To loosen the spine stand with your legs slightly apart and, letting your trunk completely relax, lean forward as far as you can. When you are down (bending from the waist) bounce the spine gently up and down, reaching down a little further each time. Don't stretch or strain, but after a short time you will find that your spine and hips become supple enough for you to touch the floor and eventually lay your palms flat on the floor.

e: Lie face down on the floor and pushing down with your hands, curve your back, putting your head back as far as it will go, so that you make a letter 'C' with your body. This will give you a complete spinal stretch. Then come forward onto your knees, like a cat, and let your spine curve in the opposite direction, so that you arch it like a cat. Put your head right down when you arch and right back when you curve. This will make the spine very flexible and supple.

f: Sitting down with your legs wide apart and your hands on the floor in front to support you, try and lift your heels as high off the floor as you can. Change the positions of your hands, move them further away from the body, and see how long you can keep your heels off the floor.

Relaxation exercise. After any exercise session, however vigorous, or even after a couple of hours gardening or housework, it is good to do a relaxation exercise to relieve any tension in the muscles.

Lie flat on the floor, on your back, with the palms of your hands facing upwards. Tense all the muscles in your feet, squeeze your toes together, and then let them relax. Tighten your calf muscles, your thighs, and squeeze your buttocks together, and then let them relax. Working your way up the body from your feet to your head, tighten each muscle and then let it go, don't forget your fingers, your shoulders, neck, mouth, eyes, nose, and scalp.

By the time you reach the end you should be totally relaxed. All your limbs will feel heavy, as if you are going to sink into the floor. After a few minutes, sit up slowly, don't rush, then stand up and have a good stretch, shake each limb separately. You will feel full of energy, and fit for anything!

Chapter Four

What Kind of Exercise?

Exercise should be fun. If you don't enjoy doing it and find it a mental strain, especially a set exercise routine, then it is important to find a method of getting the body fit that you *will* enjoy doing. Exercise does not have to be all press-ups and muscle contractions; participation in a sport of some kind is one of the best methods of getting fit, for not only is it enjoyable to do but you meet lots of people socially, make new friends, and keep healthy at the same time.

Obviously it is important to pick your sport wisely, one that you know you will enjoy and that you are physically capable of doing. Never force yourself or your children into something they really don't want to do. I saw it so many years ago, when I was a kid boxing, there were kids who used to box because their fathers wanted them to. You could tell the son hated boxing and had been pushed into it, he would never be any good at it because he didn't enjoy what he was doing. If my kids had shown any interest in boxing I would have encouraged them, but they didn't so I never pushed them. In fact they were more interested in cricket!

It is important in all sports that you never strain yourself. If you know you have a weak back, then don't participate in a sport that will put extra strain on your back muscles. Sport is important because it raises your spirits mentally too, and often that is just as essential as physical harmony in the body. In this section we will be looking at the various sports there are in this country, most of which have clubs and societies that you can join. Contact your Local Recreation Department or Citizen's Advice Bureau who will tell you where your nearest centre is. Two of the most popular sports today are ones that you don't have to join a club or society to participate in, in fact you can do it alone or let the whole family join in, and they are JOGGING and SWIMMING.

These are two useful sports for keeping fit because you can do them anywhere, and if you want to swim there is sure to be a pool within a few miles of your home. I swim for about eight months of the year, but with indoor pools there is no reason why you shouldn't swim all the year round. If you are really out of condition then swimming or jogging is advisable because they are non-competitive sports; you simply do as much as you want to do. Let's take a closer look at these two sports in greater detail . . .

The Gentle Art of Jogging

Jogging not only makes you feel great, but it is one of the most natural and effective ways of exercising the heart and lungs. Jogging is running free and easy at a comfortable trot. There is no urgency, no strain, and no competition.

The idea is to jog along at a pace that makes you no more than moderately breathless. If you do it long and often enough, in gradually increasing sessions, it will soon build up the stamina of your heart and lungs, and strengthen your leg muscles. The steady, easy rhythm of jogging will help to massage away mental and physical tension and lift depression. The joy of jogging is that virtually anyone can do it, young or old. You can do it anywhere or anytime.

How often? How much? As with any other heart and lung exercise, you will benefit most if you jog as often as possible, preferably every day. But if you can't manage that, every other day is often enough. But if you do it any less than that you will lose the training effect.

How much depends upon your state of fitness. The most important thing is to build up your jogging very gradually week by week, as with all exercises. This will give your heart, lungs and circulation time to develop the necessary stamina. As you get fitter you should be spending at least ten to twenty minutes a day jogging.

When? The best time of the day to jog is whatever time suits *you* best. Perhaps you would prefer to jog before breakfast when the air is fresher and the streets are quieter. Or you may prefer early evening before supper, when it is dark and you can't be seen by your friends! It depends on how you feel and what your other plans are, but there are certain times of the day when you must NOT jog:

* Don't jog within two hours of your last meal.
* Don't jog if you feel weak, tired, or flaked-out.
* Don't jog if you have a cold or feel one coming on.
* Don't jog in fog.

Remember. If you jog in the dark, always wear light-coloured kit so that you can easily be seen by fast moving traffic. Better still, wear something reflective.

What about the weather? Never jog in really hot weather when the sun is right overhead as this could easily give you sunstroke. If it begins to rain then press on, if it is only a shower, otherwise it is common sense to shelter. Always beware of ice in the winter.

Where? You can jog virtually anywhere you like, but preferably away from harmful diesel and exhaust fumes. If you prefer to jog on soft ground, try the park or a country path or bridleway. Or get permission to use the local school playing field or local authority sports ground. Don't be tempted to sprint downhill during the first few weeks as it is likely to cause muscle strain.

Jogger's togs. The main thing is to be comfortable and not wear any restrictive clothing. Obviously it depends on the weather, but try to wear loose-fitting and lightweight clothing. Natural fibre (such as cotton) is much better than nylon or terylene as you won't get so hot and sticky. If you are too hot you will get exhausted much quicker; if you're too cold you may stiffen and get cramp. So wear a warm top that you can take off and sling around your waist when you start to warm up. A track-suit is tailor-made for the job. In cold weather be sure to keep your head warm with a hat, few people realise that much of your body heat is lost through the top of your head.

What footwear? Wearing the correct footgear is vital. If you have an old pair of gym shoes that are broken in, but not broken up, then they will be ideal. If you have to buy a new pair of shoes then look out for the following points:

a: Make sure they have a thick cushioned rubber insole, especially at the heel.
b: Beware of protruding stitches on the inside which may cause blisters.
c: Avoid shoes with plastic linings that don't let your feet breathe.
d: Avoid shoes with high tabs at the back which will cut into your heel.
e: Choose a shoe with a good arch support.
f: Buy a size larger than your normal street shoes, if you wear thicker socks, as your feet may 'spread' a little when you jog.
g: Always break in your new shoes around the house for a couple of days before you start jogging in them.

How to start. As with all exercise, start gently and don't rush into it, especially if you are over thirty-five, unfit, overweight or a smoker. Build up gradually day by day. You should always be well within your capability. If you feel flaked-out, you've definitely overdone it. When you start, begin by walking a little way, then jogging, then walking, and so on. You should always be able to hold an ordinary conversation as you jog without being breathless. Gradually you can build it up so that you spend more time jogging than walking. If you can, go with a friend or other members of your family, as it will help to pass the time.

Below are two suggested 'Build-up Schedules' that you

may wish to follow, depending which category you fall under.

Build-up Schedule A (for fairly-fit under thirty-five-year-olds):

Week 1 – Somehow do at least half-an-hour's brisk walking a day. Walk at every opportunity. Use the stairs. Get off the bus a stop or two early. Walk to the shops. Spend the whole of your jogging sessions walking briskly.

Week 2 – Start by walking for five minutes. Then jog for thirty seconds. Walk for thirty seconds, repeat ten times. Then jog for forty-five seconds, walk for forty-five seconds, repeat three times.

Week 3 – Warm-up walk five minutes. Jog one minute, walk one minute, then repeat five times. Walk five minutes.

Week 4 – Warm-up walk two minutes. Jog two minutes, walk one minute, then repeat five times. Walk two minutes.

Week 5 and thereafter – Warm-up walk one minute. Jog for three minutes, walk one minute, then repeat five times. Over the next few weeks, increase the time spent jogging and cut down the number of walking breaks until you are eventually jogging the whole twenty minutes at the end of the sixth week.

Build-up Schedule B (for not-so-fit over thirty-five-year-olds):

Week 1 – Spend a determined week walking as much as possible as described in schedule A – work up to half-an-hour's brisk walk a day.

Week 2 – Start by walking for five minutes. Jog fifteen seconds, walk fifteen seconds, then repeat five times. Walk five minutes, jog fifteen seconds, walk fifteen seconds, then repeat five times. Walk five minutes.

Week 3 – Warm-up walk five minutes. Jog thirty seconds, walk thirty seconds, then repeat three times. Walk four minutes. Then jog thirty seconds, walk thirty seconds, then repeat three times. Walk five minutes.

Week 4 – Warm-up walk five minutes. Jog one minute, walk one minute, then repeat twice. Walk two minutes. Jog one minute, walk one minute, then repeat twice. Walk five minutes.

Week 5 – Warm-up walk five minutes. Jog one minute, walk one minute, then repeat five times. Walk five minutes.

Week 6 – Warm-up walk two minutes. Jog two minutes, walk one minute, then repeat five times. Walk two minutes.

Weeks 7 & 8 – Gradually increase the time spent jogging and cut down the number of walking breaks, until by the end of the eighth week you are jogging for ten to twelve minutes at a stretch, depending upon your level of comfort.

In the Swim

Swimming is one of the best all-round exercises, ideal for developing the three S's – stamina, suppleness and strength. The swimming pool will give you that sense of freedom, and moving through the water is certainly very soothing and relaxing, almost like a massage, so that all your worries will just melt away and you will feel fresher and fitter.

Because your body is supported by the water, your spine and joints can move freely, and there is no strain on your back, or limbs. This makes swimming especially beneficial for elderly people, for the obese and for anyone with back trouble, arthritis or rheumatism.

If you only normally swim in the summer whilst on holiday, then take things easily to start with. Don't go mad and swim six lengths of the pool just to prove you can do it.

A length of a bath is usually around twenty-five metres, and much further than it looks – so work in widths Concentrate on a good stretch and streamlined body position. Swim with a smooth, easy, relaxed stroke. Take deep breaths in time with the action, and don't swim so hard that you tire yourself.

Try a variety of styles – breaststroke, backstroke, etc. That way you exercise different groups of muscles and joints. For example: the breaststroke is great for the hips and knees, the backstroke and crawl for the shoulders and trunk. But you should avoid the butterfly stroke if you suffer from any back trouble.

It is best to build up slowly to two or three twenty minute sessions a week. Or daily if you really take to it. Virtually all pools are heated and most are indoors, so it is an easy all-weather way to keep fit.

Admission to municipal pools is quite cheap. Many open early on one or two mornings a week – so how about a dip before work? Or go at the end of a tiring day, to unwind. They usually have a few evening sessions each week.

Before you swim, remember these four points:
  * Never swim within two hours of a heavy meal.
  * Don't let yourself get too cold, or you may get cramp.
  * If swimming in the sea, don't swim where there are dangerous currents or tides.
  * Don't be put off if you can't swim. You can get lessons at your local pool. There are classes for all ages and, if you prefer it, private tuition can usually be arranged.

As with many sports, remember you are never too old to learn. No matter how unfit you are, as long as you take things easy at the start and gradually work your way to fitness there is no reason why you shouldn't attempt any sport you wish. Obviously you won't end up with an Adonis physique, but you will feel fit to cope with your daily life.

Jogging and swimming are two of the more popular sporting activities in this country. Let us, however, have a brief look at some of the other leisure pursuits that you can participate in. Some are sports that you can play on your own, such as golf, but some are team games where it will be necessary for you to join a local club. With luck you will find, in this group, an activity which will suit you. It is a fun way of keeping fit and will help you to relax too.

Archery:

Not such a popular sport as it used to be, but a marvellous exercise for the arm muscles and for your concentration too. Obviously good eyesight is necessary, but no special clothes are needed except a leather glove to protect your hands. This is one activity which you must join a club to learn, don't just get a bow and arrow and try and practice on your own as this could have highly dangerous results. Arrows can be lethal, look what happened to King Harold!

Arrows come in different sizes and weights, so do the bows, so varying degrees of strength are required to pull the arrow back. Olympic champions pull up to forty-two pounds in pressure to release their arrows, which can be aimed at targets up to 300 feet away.

Badminton:

As with tennis, this can be played as a singles or doubles game, but you will find the racket much lighter. As with archery, it is a good sport for strengthening muscles and increasing your co-ordination and concentration – especially good for strengthening the wrist muscles. The game can be very strenuous so beginners should take things easy at first. Experts have been known to send the shuttlecock across the net at over 100 mph so once you become more fit and experienced it can be an exciting way of burning up those excess calories.

There are clubs and societies all over the country, and you may find that a local college or institute has an evening class for beginners. You will, however, need special clothing to play – usually white tennis clothes and plimsolls will be required, especially on an indoor court.

Bowling:

There are two types of bowling, the kind we usually associate with Sir Francis Drake which is played on a beautiful smooth green, and ten-pin bowling where you attempt to knock down as many pins as you can. Both games are excellent for keeping the spine supple and strengthening your arms. A good exercise for older people because it is not too energetic.

Ten-pin bowling can be found in many towns, you don't need to be a club member and it is quite inexpensive. All the family can play too so it really turns into a social occasion, and if there is no bowling alley nearby then you can just as easily play at home on the lawn with the kids' skittles!

Outdoor bowling is a little more specialised and takes greater skill as you have to get your bowl as near as you can to the white jack, and because the bowls are weighted on one side it takes a little practice to know which direction to roll them and how much force to apply. Soft shoes are essential so as not to damage the green. A very peaceful and relaxing game, for someone who prefers the quieter sports.

Finally, there are smaller, lighter bowls available which are known as 'Carpet bowls'. These can be played indoors if you have a large enough room to play in. These are quite expensive to buy, but are usually beautifully finished and will last a lifetime if treated with respect. The game is exactly the same as outdoor bowls, but can obviously be played in all weathers.

Boxing:

I couldn't deal with sporting activities without saying something about this one! Obviously I could write a whole book on this subject, but without being biased this really is an excellent activity for keeping fit.

It is advisable to join a boxing club to learn, but if you have a weak heart or poor eyesight this is not to be recommended. Gloves are essential, of course, and should weigh at least twelve ounces for beginners. A great activity for learning self-discipline, building up your leg and arm muscles, and strengthening your heart and lungs. At a boxing club you will probably begin training with a punch-bag, and this is a great way to practice at home too. As you become experienced you will be matched up with a boxer of your own weight. So if you're five foot tall don't worry that you'll have to box against someone who's six-foot two!

Cricket:

This is a summer team game for which it will be necessary to join a cricket club if you wish to play properly, although there is no reason why you shouldn't have a family game in the garden and get just as much exercise. Not such an energetic game as it looks because you do relatively little running, but you do have to have good concentration and co-ordination, and your arm muscles will gradually strengthen. To play in a team you will need suitable white protective pads and clothing which can be very expensive. You will probably get more exercise in a family game, but if you do play at home, use a softer ball as a hard cricket ball can be lethal.

Cycling:

An activity that you can indulge in on your own or with friends. Excellent for increasing the strength and mobility of your legs, and building up the stamina of your heart and lungs. Good for people with bad feet or arthritis because you don't have to bear weight on your feet. Try cycling to work, it's much cheaper than the bus and you can usually avoid the worst of the traffic jams. Do make sure you signal clearly and can see and be seen at all times. Safety is most important, so remember:

* Always be sure that you can be seen easily at night. Keep your front and rear lights in good working order, and don't forget to switch them on. Wear light-coloured clothing or a reflective jacket.

* Beware of careless traffic, especially in towns. Drivers tend to have a nasty habit of cutting corners without a thought for the cyclist on the inside.

* Don't change lanes unexpectedly or weave in and out of slow-moving traffic. Take the very greatest care when turning right.

* Always give clear hand signals. Learn the Highway Code before you start.

Cycling in the country is sheer pleasure. Quiet lanes, clean air, birds singing. But beware of fast drivers, and if with friends, cycle in single file on busy or narrow roads. Look out for your local cycle club and make new friends too.

Dancing:

If a boisterous sport is not your idea of fun, then try an activity like dancing. There are many types of dance class all over the country from ballet to country dancing. Whatever the type, whether ballroom or disco, dancing is a good all-round exercise as it stretches every muscle in the body. It is important that you wear good shoes that are flexible but will support your feet too. As you progress you will gain more stamina and become supple. Classes are a good way of meeting people and it can become a social occasion too. There is also no reason why you shouldn't practice at home. It really is a fun way of keeping fit, whatever your age or sex.

Fencing:

If you think you are another Errol Flynn then why not join a fencing club. You may find it expensive at first because it is *essential* that you have all the protective clothing, from the face mask to the padded suit. Your local club will give you details of where this can be obtained, and may even be able to supply it. This is a very graceful sport, and is superb for movement and co-ordination, which is why so many actors learn fencing at drama school.

Football:

Probably one of the most popular sports in this country. It can be played anywhere at any time, whether it is on the beach, in the park, in the snow. In fact as long as you have a ball you can play football. If you wish, you can join a local team or club, but just kicking a ball around with a few friends will keep you in trim in exactly the same way. It's great fun to play with the kids too. If you are on your own, then find a suitable wall without windows and doors in it, and kick a ball against it. This will strengthen your leg muscles, and your heart and lungs will benefit too.

Golf:

One of my favourite sports this. There is sure to be a club near to you where a professional coach will teach you how to play, and a few lessons are very worthwhile to beginners so that you know how to stand, how to hold the club, and so on. It is necessary to know exactly how to hit the ball, although it seems like common sense. The ball will go much further with a light tap in the right place than it will with a good hard slam. Not a very physically demanding sport, but a healthy one because it involves the use of a great many muscles, requires concentration, a great deal of walking which will increase the circulation and so strengthen your heart a little. There is plenty of fresh air too. Clubs can be bought or hired at the golf club. Beginners may like to visit a driving-range where they will be given a bucket of about fifty balls to practise their shots. Whatever your age this really is an ideal sport for keeping yourself healthy.

Gymnastics:

A sport for anyone, although it is advisable to be in reasonable condition when starting. Find a gymnasium where you will be given expert guidance, otherwise you could seriously damage your muscles. The advantage of a gymnasium is the variety of equipment available, from trampolines to ropes, which are a really fun way of keeping fit. You will require soft gym shoes and a leotard, or shorts and a T-shirt. Every muscle in the body will be used.

Horse Riding:

This is one of the oldest sports known to man. There are many riding-schools around the country which will teach you how to ride correctly. It is a good exercise for posture and balance as a great deal of muscle power has to be used. It is essential that you have the correct gear too, especially a proper riding hat that will protect your head if you fall as even the most experienced riders fall off at times! Treat your horse with respect and don't underestimate its strength. If you find that horse-riding really is your forte, after a few years you can turn it into a competitive sport by show jumping, dressage, or cross-country riding. If out on your own, keep away from main roads, and try and stick to paths that are marked for horse riders.

Skating:

Another fun sport this. There are two types: Ice skating and roller skating. Ice skating uses a lot of energy and so burns up the calories. Be sure to go to a proper skating rink, and never skate on a pond or river that has ice on it. At the rink you will be fitted out with proper skates, but take the greatest care if you have weak ankles as these can so easily be twisted whilst skating. Wear thick, warm, and protective clothing too, as you are sure to end up flat on your back!

Roller skating is not just for children, and has become very popular again. Choose your skates carefully so that they are a perfect fit, and if possible skate at a proper roller rink. If you must skate elsewhere avoid pavements and roads, but stick to parks and surfaces specially designed for skating. Again wear protective clothing, otherwise you might end up with a few bruises, and most important of all – look out for other people, you could easily knock someone over if you are not careful.

Rowing:

A sport which can involve the whole family. Rowing boats and canoes can often be hired on rivers, but it might be wise to join a rowing club first to gain initial training in rowing technique. Do not take up rowing unless you are a competent swimmer, and even if you are always wear a life-jacket. Wear waterproof clothing, and make sure it is warm too. Most important of all – tell someone where you are going and when you intend to be back.

Rugby:

A very strenuous game, and quite rough too. There are two types, Rugby League which is both amateur and professional, and Rugby Union, which is an amateur game. As this involves a lot of exercise all the muscles are strengthened, although it is necessary to be relatively fit before taking it up. It is best to join a Rugby Club, as it is not really a family game that anyone can play.

Skiing:

Not a sport that you can participate in very much in this country. There are some slopes in Scotland, and some of the larger sports centres do have dry ski slopes. If you take a holiday to a country like Switzerland, you may get an opportunity to ski, but do have professional instruction first. Do some limbering-up exercises before you begin, and wear several layers of protective, warm clothing. Boots should be particularly sturdy and well-fitting. If you are a beginner, start with short skis rather than long ones. This exercise will make your leg muscles strong, and burn up a lot of calories too.

Squash:

An increasingly popular sport in this country, although not advisable for someone who is really out of condition or who has a weak heart. It requires an enormous amount of energy, but has the advantage of being a game which you can practice on your own. Wear clothes that you would wear on a tennis court. Have some professional coaching at first so that you learn the correct strokes. A particularly good game for concentration, co-ordination, strengthening muscles, and increasing stamina.

Tennis:

If you have never played tennis before, start off in a doubles match as you will find it easier. It is purely a matter of personal preference whether or not you play on a hard or soft court. Many prefer a grass court because it slows the ball down very slightly. In the summer during Wimbledon fortnight watch as much tennis as you can and look out for the varying styles and techniques. A great deal can be learnt from watching experts in action. A tennis racket is heavier than a squash or badminton racket, so take great care of the wrist, and wear an elastic bandage around it for support if you feel you may have trouble. To keep in shape it will be necessary to play throughout the summer. White tennis gear is available from all sports shops, and choose your racket carefully – some are a lot lighter than others, especially the lightweight steel framed rackets.

Volleyball:

A popular team game in which a lightweight ball is thrown or hit across a net approximately eight feet high with the hands. It firms up leg and arm muscles, and is an ideal sport for ladies to play as it is not too boisterous. It is also an ideal family game and can be played on the beach or in the garden. Make sure that the ball is not too heavy as it can seriously injure your wrist – it might be wise to invest in a proper volleyball.

Walking:

As long as you have some comfortable walking shoes you can participate in one of the healthiest outdoor activities available. You can go as fast or as slow as you wish, in your own time. It will do wonders for your circulation, it will firm up the muscles, burn up the calories, improve your breathing, and make you feel glowing and full of health. It also aids digestion, and will help you sleep at night.

Water Skiing:

This always looks very dangerous, but in fact it is quite easy and even children or handicapped people can participate. Before joining a skiing club, see if they will let you have a trial lesson, just to make sure you really like it. It is important that you always wear a life-jacket, and avoid all obstacles, especially swimmers! It will help strengthen your leg and arm muscles and really is a fun exercise, but do have professional training.

Weight-Lifting:

Believe it or not, this activity is just as popular with women as with men, because it helps pull in your muscles and give you that perfect figure you've always dreamed of. If you want a body like a Greek God then have a go at weight-lifting. Always have a qualified instructor so that you lift the weights correctly, and be certain to do some limbering-up exercises first so that your muscles are warm before you start. It is a very vigorous exercise and should be done at least twice a week to build up your muscles. Contrary to most forms of exercise, it is not advisable to start too lightly if you want to build up strength. Some experts claim that if you pick up light weights, say ten times, you will feel exhausted, but if you start with something quite heavy, say eighty pounds, you will find that you can pick up lighter weights quite easily without being exhausted. Obviously you need professional guidance, and it is not wise to pick up too much too soon. Your instructor will advise you. Development of muscles will be much quicker if you train often for short periods rather than one long training session a week. Increase the weights pound by pound as you progress.

Whatever your interest or sport, remember the key attitude is to have fun and enjoy yourself. You will not get fit if it is a mental strain to participate in something you don't like in the hope that it will do you good. I keep fit these days by playing golf and swimming, which I love. From ten years old, I have been in gymnasiums. Until I was twenty-seven I sweated in gyms, and I said after that I just want to get out into some fresh air and walk around the golf course. So if there is something you really enjoy, then get out there and do it. If you've always had a burning ambition to go horse riding or water-skiing, well now's the time to start. It's never too soon – or too late.

Chapter Five

Useful Exercise Aids

As you look around your home you may not realise that there are many everyday, household items that can be very useful to you in your exercise routines. Exercise aids will help improve your mobility, strength and muscle power. Here are just a few exercise aids that you should find in most homes:

Broom Handle (or a piece of cane or bamboo):

Any old walking stick or broom handle can become a useful piece of exercising apparatus. A couple of exercises in which you will find it is a help is in the 'sit-up' exercise, where you lie flat on your back and sit up from the waist upwards, keeping your legs firmly on the floor. If you lie on your back with your arms straight up in the air in front of you, hold the broom handle in your hands and use it as a balance to pull yourself up.

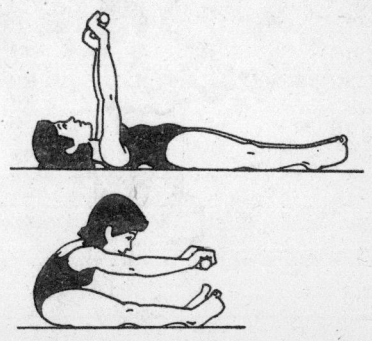

A variation on touching your toes is to put the broom handle about eight inches in front of your toes and bend over from the waist to pick it up, without bending the knees.

To exercise your arms, abdominal muscles, and check your breathing, put the broom handle on the floor, and lie down on your back so that the broom is about two feet from your head. Breathe in and keeping your spine flat on the ground (and your head) reach your arms into the air and over your head and stretch until you can grasp the broom. Breathing out, lift the handle above your head and forward to rest on your tummy. Breathe out and replace it in its original position. Repeat five to ten times, depending upon your fitness. Remember to keep the spine as flat on the floor as you can.

To strengthen your wrists and fingers, tie a piece of string around the centre of your broom, make sure the string is about four to five feet long and quite strong. To the other end of the rope or string, attach a weight of some kind, say approximately five pounds. Extend your arms in front of you, holding the broom handle, and twist it so that you winch the weight up, then lower it slowly. As your wrists become stronger you can increase the weight on the end.

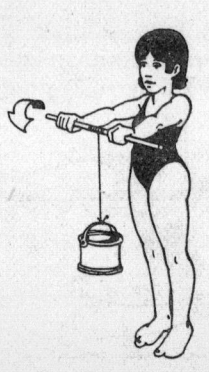

Place the broom handle at the back of your neck and your hands grasping each side. Now do various spinal bends to the right and left, forwards and backwards, keeping the broom in place on your shoulders.

Leg Strengtheners:

There are a variety of household objects that can be used to strengthen your legs. Take, for example, a bag of shopping which is not *too* heavy. Sit on a table and hook the handle of the bag over your ankle. Straighten your leg as high as you can, pointing the toes at the same time, lifting the shopping bag as high as you can. Alternate each leg. If you have knee trouble, don't try this exercise. Consult your doctor first.

Lying on your back, with toes pointed, place a fairly heavy book on your feet. Keeping your back firmly on the floor, lift your feet slowly and as high as you can without the book falling off. If you find a book is too heavy or uncomfortable, try the same exercise with a heavy cushion or pillow. You can do a similar exercise by lying on your back and placing a cushion between your feet and, making sure that your knees are touching, lift the cushion up as high as you can. The object should be to try and lift the cushion right over your head and place it there, slowly returning your feet to their original position. You will feel a very strong pull on your tummy muscles at the same time, so don't do it too often to start with as otherwise you will find your abdomen very stiff the following day.

Toe Strengtheners:

Take off your shoes and socks and place a pencil on the floor about six inches away. Reach out with your foot and try and pick up the pencil with your toes. Try it with each foot ten times. Do this daily and you will find that your feet will become more supple.

When you have mastered the art of picking up pencils,

try putting the pencil an inch further away each day so that you have to stretch more. If you replace the pencil with a marble, you may find that much more difficult.

Whenever possible walk around the house in your bare feet as this will really let them breathe. Keep them scrupulously clean, bathe them regularly in salt water, and pay particular attention to your shoes. Ill-fitting shoes can damage your feet for life. As your toes become really strong, attempt to pick up various objects with them, such as cotton-reels, a string of beads, a matchbox, and so on. Pick up an object with each foot at the same time – this will take real concentration. To exercise the whole foot, pick up larger objects, such as a balloon, or a ball of wool, placing them between the soles of your two feet. As you get older your feet become less supple so it is essential to keep them mobile by doing exercises such as these, they will not only remain flexible but will aid your circulation too.

If you do have any problems with your feet, visit a state registered chiropodist as soon as possible; if you take good care of your feet this should not be necessary. Always change your shoes at least twice a day, and socks or stockings daily. If your feet tend to perspire, then dust them with talcum, or a special foot powder.

Screwed-up Newspaper:

Yes, believe it or not, a ball of newspaper can be used as an exercise aid.

To strengthen the arms and chest, stand straight, with your legs slightly apart and your elbows up and out at shoulder height. Hold the newspaper between both your hands, about six inches away from you, and squeeze it as hard as you can. Relax and repeat it ten times.

If you have arthritis or rheumatism in your fingers, a ball of newspaper to squeeze between the fingers will help strengthen the muscles.

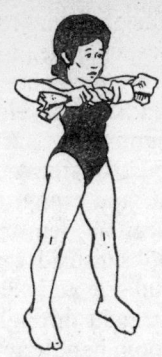

Briefcase:

A briefcase full of books can be used as an aid. Simply stand erect with your legs slightly apart. Keeping your spine straight, lean to the right and pick up the briefcase in your right hand and slowly straighten yourself into an upright position. Hold for a count of ten and slowly replace the bag on the floor. Replace, and repeat with your left hand. As you become fitter you can increase the weight of the case by adding more books.

Sugar:

Bags of sugar are a useful aid because you know exactly how much they weigh, and therefore what weight you are carrying.

Place a bag of sugar on either side of you. Stand with your legs apart between the two bags and, bending your knees, come down into a squat position. Take a bag of sugar in each hand and keeping your spine straight, your head upright and looking in front of you, come slowly up to a standing position. As you become fitter you can carefully raise the bags above your head and hold for a count of five, before bending the knees and lowering yourself down again to replace the bags on the floor. If you find sugar too heavy at first, then use two tins of soup, or tins of baked beans! – whatever weight you feel capable of lifting. If you feel any strain on your back at all, then abandon the exercise.

A good exercise for ladies to develop the bust is to hold a bag of sugar in each hand with your arms out at shoulder height in front of you. Breathing in, swing your arms outwards. Breathe out, and swing them in again to their original position. Repeat this ten times. If you find sugar too heavy, then use books instead, but make sure that both your books are of equal size and weight. Keep your head erect and your spine straight throughout.

With the aid of a broom handle and a couple of weights, you can make your own bar bells to do similar exercises. If you take a rod or broom handle and screw two cup hooks, one at either end, you can hang small bags of marbles, sugar, pebbles, etc, on the ends to use in weight training.

Door Frames:

If you have a sturdy and strong door frame in your home with a wooden surround you can use it to exercise yourself, but take great care not to damage yourself or the property.

Stand in the doorway, so that when you stretch your arms out you have one hand in each room. Reach up and grasp the surround at the top of the door and try and pull yourself up with your arms and lift your feet off the floor. Once you become really strong you can do an exercise whereby you raise yourself up putting your head in the left hand room, then lower yourself down. Now raise yourself up, putting your head in the right hand room. Repeat.

A good stretching exercise is to stand in an open doorway with your legs slightly apart. Reach up and push against the top of the doorway with your hands and downwards with your feet at the same time so that you have a really good stretch.

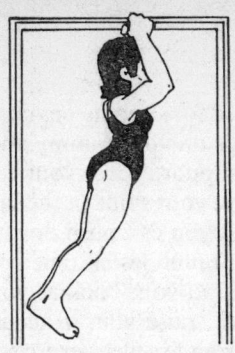

Likewise, if it is wide enough, stand in the doorway facing into the room with your feet pressed into the bottom right and left hand corners. Reach up as high as you can trying to put your hands into the top right and left hand corners, so that your body is making a star-shape, and push with your hands and feet as though you were trying to push the doorway apart. Imagine that you are standing in a narrow alleyway with a high wall to your right and left and the walls are slowly closing in on you – you must push as hard as you can to keep them apart.

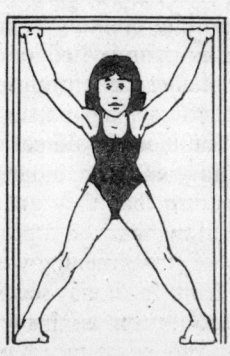

Bed:

This is not to be used for sleeping on, but as an exercise aid!
Lie face downwards on your tummy and hook your heels
under the bed as a support. Raise your head back to look at
the ceiling and curve your spine at the same time. To make
things easier at first you can push down on the floor with
your hands. As your muscles become stronger, grasp your
hands together behind your back as you do this exercise,
and as you go back, raise your arms as high as you can
behind you. This is an excellent exercise for the spine and
your posture, but if you feel any pain in your back stop
immediately.

As you look around your house you will discover more
items that can be used as household aids, but obviously
consider the safety aspect before you attempt any exercise.
If anything appears even the slightest bit unsteady, or too
heavy for you, then don't take the risk. The object of the
exercise is to get fit, not to end up in hospital!

Creating Your Own Gymnasium:

If you and your friends really wish to take fitness seriously
and have a spare room or empty garage, then it might be an
idea for you to consider creating your own gymnasium.
This need not be as complicated or as expensive as it
sounds, especially if there is a group of you who could
supply the equipment.

If your gymnasium is in an old garage where there are
beams, take advantage of these to hang a couple of ropes
from them. Make sure that they are perfectly safe and
secure. Climbing and swinging on ropes is not only fun, but
is also a good way of strengthening your arm and tummy
muscles. However tempting it may seem, do not slide down
the rope from top to bottom as this will burn and blister
your hands. If you buy some pieces of dowling you can

make your own rope ladder too, but make sure the wood is perfectly smooth and has no splinters in it as this could be dangerous. Varnish the wood if you can.

An exercise cycle can be made out of an old bicycle by taking off the wheels and bolting it to a piece of wood. Very old cycles are ideal for this as they are much higher off the ground. Again, make quite sure that this is perfectly secure. By sitting on it you can pedal away and exercise your thighs, calves and ankles provided, of course, that there is some resistance to the pedals.

Spread several mats around so that you can exercise on the floor. If your 'gym' is large enough, you and your family can use it to play various ball games and group exercises. On the walls you can keep charts of your progress, such as your weight, and a list of your daily exercise schedule so that you know exactly how many exercises you need to do each day.

Obviously not everyone will have the necessary space to devote to a gymnasium, but if you have, and are enthusiastic enough, there really is no end to the possibilities and the inexpensive equipment you can create to keep yourself really in top form.

Chapter Six

You Are What You Eat

It is all very well keeping yourself active and well-exercised but how can you be sure that your body is getting the right nourishment?

Did you realise that the average person swallows about *half-a-ton* of food a year? That is a lot of food, and doesn' include drink either. Your body is remarkably efficient a extracting exactly what it wants from the vast mixture tha you eat, but it can only cope up to a certain point, just a you in your daily life can only cope with a certain amoun of work. If you go on eating too much of one thing and no enough of the others, you will eventually find that you are lacking in some necessary nutrient. You will get out o condition and your health and well-being will suffer. Afte all, you really are what you eat, so think of that before you tuck into a large cream cake or trifle. It may look and tast good, but what good is it doing you?

How Do We Work?

Before we can understand why we should eat the righ foods, it is necessary to understand a little bit about how our body works. You may know, for example, how a ca engine works, and how if you don't give it oil it will seize up Well our bodies are similar to a car, for everything we take in is converted into energy. Every single thing you eat every chip and chocolate bar, is broken up by the body. The teeth chew it, the saliva moistens it, the tongue helps the food on its way to the throat where your epiglottis directs i down to your stomach.

The food first goes down the oesophagus which contract

and pushes the food down to your stomach. Your stomach is very flexible and changes its shape according to what you put in it, but at the most it holds about two-and-a-half pints. The food is churned around, mixed with gastric juices and hydrochloric acid and so breaks down into even smaller pieces. It then moves to the duodenum where it is mixed with more juices and bile from the gall bladder, and from there to the small intestine, which is over twenty feet long. Here it is chemically broken down and all the nutrients are absorbed into the bloodstream. It will take four to eight hours for this to happen. Finally it will move to the large intestine where the water will be absorbed, and what remains becomes a soft solid of indigestible remnants, waste products, and millions of bacteria. It will remain here between four to twenty-five hours when it will eventually pass out of the body.

That is a very simplified explanation of a highly complicated process, but basically we know that anything we eat will take *at least* fifteen hours to work through the system, and we know the better the quality of food we put in, the better our bodies will be at digesting the food, and the healthier we will be.

Your Own Body

Your body, the way you eat, and the sort of person you are, is unique to you. To start with, the genes inherited from your parents can determine how your body chemistry, or metabolism, reacts to and copes with particular food. The tendency to put on weight, for example, often runs in families – and if it does, it will mean that you need to take extra care.

Your parents can 'shape' you in another way too, because your upbringing will effect your basic attitude to food – like whether you have a sweet tooth, nibble between meals, take big mouthfuls or eat chips with everything. Eating habits, both good and bad, do tend to get passed on. Are you passing on sensible ones to your children?

65

Your life style, too, will be different to other people. How much time and money you spend on food, how much alcohol you drink, how much exercise you get – all these things alter the balance between food and fitness as far as calories are concerned.

Finally, your age and sex will affect this balance. For example, women are more likely than men to put on weight as they get older. So, we are all very different and it is important that you get to know yourself.

The Correct Balance for You

Your food should balance your body's need for the raw materials to build and repair your body:

NUTRIENTS such as protein, fats and carbohydrates.

ENERGY (Calories) necessary for your body to keep alive and active and for its thousands of different functions to work.

VITAMINS, MINERALS and WATER all essential for health.

FIBRE (a complex mixture of natural plant substances) we usually call it roughage, is also needed for a variety of reasons.

Today we tend to eat far too many nutrients and far too many calories, but not enough fibre, so it is essential to strike the right balance. If you eat a fairly varied diet, it is virtually impossible to go short of proteins, vitamins, and minerals. It is also more than likely that you will be eating too many fats and carbohydrates. Those who are fussy about their food or go on crash diets are the people most likely to be missing out on nutrients. But the average person is certainly getting enough nutrients.

Look at proteins, for example. On average we eat twice as much as we need. Although we need protein there is nothing to be gained by eating too much.

Likewise, vitamin pills are of little value. If you eat fresh fruit, vegetables, cereals, eggs, fish, meat, and some dairy products, you will be getting more than enough vitamins

As for minerals, if we eat liver, kidneys and green leafy vegetables, we are getting enough. Perhaps pregnant women may need extra iron, but on the whole we have more than enough for excellent health.

Fibre

Throughout man's evolution his daily diet came mainly from plants – unrefined cereals, root vegetables, fruit and nuts – meat was just an occasional delicacy. This meant that over hundreds of thousands of years our ancestors adapted to food containing a high proportion of dietary fibre. This is a complex mixture of mostly indigestible plant substances, including what we call 'roughage'.

Our diet today, in comparison to our ancestors', consists of relatively little dietary fibre. It consists mainly of meat and dairy products which contain no fibre. Also many of the bread and cereals we eat have had the fibre refined out.

Fibre is essential to the bowels, it prevents constipation, haemorrhoids, and diverticulitis. Some experts believe that lack of fibre may lead to diabetes and heart disease. Fibre is the only important item that your daily diet is likely to lack, and it can be filling and not fattening.

How to eat more fibre:

* Eat more bread, especially wholemeal. A cheap source of fibre and nutrients without concentrated calories.

* Eat more potatoes – an excellent filler, and needn't be fattening if you don't load them with butter or fry them in fat.

* Have a high-fibre cereal for breakfast. The more wheatbran it contains, the higher its fibre content.

* Have more meals based on beans, peas and lentils, using meat more sparingly.

* Green vegetables, not overcooked but just softened, are high in fibre.

* Eat plenty of fresh fruit and salads which are low in calories.

* Make room for fibre by not eating between meals.

Daily bread. On average we eat half as much bread as we did thirty years ago, most of which is white and has had the wheatbran removed. But wholemeal bread, which is unrefined, still contains all the bran and all the fibre.

Brown bread (sometimes called 'Wheatmeal') is made partly from bran and partly from refined flour. So the best to eat is 100% *wholemeal* bread – it is tastier and chewier than supermarket whitebread, and has all the original wheatbran and wheatgerm. It may cost more, but it's worth it.

Make your own bread.

Ingredients:

1lb wholemeal flour	½ oz fresh yeast
1 dessertspoon vegetable oil	1 teaspoon sugar
1 teaspoon salt	½ pt warm water

Sprinkle sugar on to yeast and stir gently. Leave to liquify while you add salt and oil to flour. Add warm water to liquified yeast. Add yeast mixture to flour, mix well. Knead and shape. Put dough into well-greased 2 lb loaf tin and leave in warm place to rise. Bake in oven 400°F (Mark 6) for 15 minutes then at 350°F (Mark 4) for another 15 minutes. Remove loaf from tin. Tap bottom of loaf with knuckles. It should sound hollow. If not, bake for a little longer.

The Energy Crisis

Nearly all that we eat contains energy – measured as calories; the higher the calorie rating, the more energy. But don't be fooled into thinking that the more calories you eat the more energetic you will be. Unfortunately your body doesn't work like that. You need to balance the amount of energy in your diet with the amount of energy you are going o use, because if you eat more than you use this surplus nergy becomes stored as FAT. This is a big problem!

If you are overweight, there is a long list of difficulties, lisadvantages and diseases that are liable to trouble you. From ordinary everyday things like difficulty in getting lothes to fit, difficulty getting about, awkwardness, mbarrassment, even marital disharmony and serious problems like shortness of breath, varicose veins, foot rouble, backache, arthritis, chest trouble, gallstones, high lood pressure, diabetes, heart attacks and strokes!

To make matters even worse, if that is possible, overweight people are more likely to be accident victims, to have difficult pregnancies, and to suffer complications after an operation. So take a serious look at yourself now.

Are You Overweight?:

You may not realise it, but almost half the population of this country is overweight. This means there is a fifty-fifty hance that you are a fatty. No, don't argue, just try this little test . . .

* Do you have difficulty squeezing into your old clothes? That's fat!
* Stand naked in front of a full-length mirror and bob up and down. Does your flesh joggle like a jelly? That's fat!
* Pinch the skin at the back of your upper arm, halfway between your shoulder and your elbow. Is the fold of skin more than about an inch thick? That's very fat!

Check your weight too and see if it is consistent with our build and frame. If you are overweight, you should weigh yourself regularly.

* Weigh yourself once a week. Not oftener than that.
* Use the same scales each time.
* Wear the same amount of clothing – or better, none at all.
* Always weigh at the same time of day to avoid twenty-our hour fluctuations.

69

* Stand evenly on the scales – don't lean forwards or backwards.
* Keep a note of your weight.
* And make sure you stay slim!

Cut the Fat!

The average person in Britain today eats far too much fatty food, and instead of getting energy from the fibre foods we rely too much on food from animals. Meat and dairy produce contain a great deal of fat. Bacon and cheese are particularly fatty and some cream cheeses are nearly 50% fat, so pick your cheese carefully:

Cheese	Fat Content
Cottage Cheese	4%
Cheese Spread	23%
Edam Cheese	23%
Camembert Cheese	23%
Processed Cheese	25%
Danish Blue type	29%
Cheddar Cheese	34%
Stilton Cheese	40%
Cream Cheese	47%

Any fatty food has a high concentration of calories especially things like butter. With fat, you only have to eat a little more than you need and the surplus calories turn themselves into instant fat on you!

Apart from becoming overweight, another very good reason for cutting down on fat may be the most important - your heart.

Heart disease is the biggest killer in the Western world.

The problem starts when fatty substances collect inside the blood vessels. This makes them narrower and finally may block them altogether. What we eat can make a difference and most doctors agree that by reducing the amount of fat in our food, we can prevent this happening.

The best advice is to cut down on the total amount of fat you eat, especially animal and dairy fats, but don't replace them with plant fats, such as vegetable oils.

Here's how to avoid too much fatty food:

* Cut down on butter and margarine. Don't cut out bread, but eat thicker slices spread with less margarine or butter.
* Go easy on cakes, pastries and biscuits, which are rich in fat as well as sugar.
* Chocolate, whether plain or milk, is nearly one-third fat.
* Eat more vegetable-based dishes. Boiled or baked potatoes, rice, beans, peas and lentils. That gives you less fat and more fibre.
* Eat fish more often. Especially white fish, but not in thick batter!
* Choose leaner cuts of meat and cut off any fatty bits.
* Chicken has less fat than any other meat and is usually cheaper.
* Say no to cream. Double dairy is nearly half fat. Try natural yoghurt instead. And try skimmed milk.
* Have less fried food, as they all have huge quantities of fat. Grill rather than fry.

A Spoonful of Sugar?

Do you take sugar in tea or coffee? If you do, you may not realise that the average British adult consumes nearly a hundredweight (43 Kg or 95 lb) of sugar every year. Sugar (sucrose) is a highly concentrated form of energy. That annual sackful contains enough energy to keep you walking briskly for over two thousand miles!

Obviously we don't need it all. It's nice of course, and a very quick source of energy if you really need it – but most people don't. It is so easy to eat too much sugar and

71

overload yourself with calories. Not only are you likely to get fat, but you also run a great risk of losing your teeth through sugar-induced dental decay.

Sugar is a standard ingredient in many foods. Apart from obvious things like sweets, preserves, cakes, pastries and biscuits, it is also in syrups of tinned fruit, savoury sauces and many sweetened drinks.

So, if you know you are taking too much sugar, and many of us are, try and gradually wean yourself off it. Start by taking less in your tea and coffee, cutting down by, say, half-a-spoonful every fortnight, until you're off it altogether. You'll find this far easier than just suddenly stopping it. You will also start to notice all sorts of other subtler flavours in your food, previously blotted out by sweetness. If you find that you really can't do without the taste, at least substitute saccharine whenever you can. It is sweeter than sugar and calorie-free.

A Pinch of Salt

When you are cooking, try using a little less sugar than the recipe suggests, and salt too. Replace it with spices and herbs. You will find that you can greatly reduce the amount of sugar in cakes without really noticing it and, by using less salt in your cooking, you will be able to taste the food itself. We tend to eat about ten times more salt a day than we actually need. So try tasting the food itself, and avoid overpowering the taste with sugar and salt. You'll enjoy your food more and feel a lot better for it too.

Daily Vitamins

Vitamins are essential to our diet and are found in small quantities in our food. They help protect us against illness and disease, and are important to our general health. Our diet today tends to provide us with an adequate amount of vitamins, and very few people today are lacking.

The body does, however, need only a certain amount of vitamins and there is nothing to gain by having too many,

o as long as you have a sensible and varied diet you should
e receiving sufficient for your requirements. In fact it is
ossible to be ill through having too much of the fat soluble
itamins, so if you are taking drops or tablets containing
itamins A and D stick to the recommended dose.

Vitamin A	Important in children for the formation of healthy teeth and bones. It is found in dairy products such as milk and eggs, and in fish, such as halibut.
Vitamin B	Contains fifteen different substances, including Thiamin, Riboflavin, and Niacin, and is necessary for our nerves, vision, digestion, and formation of red blood cells. Found in food containing wheatgerm and yeast.
Vitamin C	Contrary to popular belief, there is no conclusive evidence that vitamin C prevents colds. However it does control the formation of teeth and bones, and red blood cells, and ensures correct healing of broken bones and wounds. It is found in fresh fruit, especially citrus fruit, and vegetables, but is quickly destroyed by cooking.
Vitamin D	Important to the digestive system, and is essential for retaining calcium in the bones. It is found in cod liver oil and dairy products.
Vitamin E	This helps in the healing of the skin, and might also be connected with fertility, although there is no definite evidence to prove this fact. It is found in spinach, wheatgerm, watercress, and lettuce.
Vitamin K	This is necessary for the blood to clot when you cut yourself, and is found mainly in green vegetables such as cabbage and spinach.

The River of Life:

Few people realise the most vital and important part of our diet – water. It is something we all take for granted, but it is one of the most essential elements of the body. Our bodies are actually two-thirds water and it has many important functions. If it came to the worst, a person could survive for some time without vitamins and other basic nutrients, but only a few days without water.

Water contains traces of minerals, and a lack of it will slow up the body's metabolism. We are almost totally dependent upon water so it is important to drink plenty of fluid daily to keep your kidneys and other internal organs in perfect working order. Much of our food contains a high percentage of water, and our body tells us of its need by making us thirsty. If you have ever wondered about thirst you will have realised that it is more than just a dryness of the mouth, otherwise your first mouthful of drink would be sufficient. Instead we get a feeling of thirst when the body feels it requires more water, especially during hot weather when a high percentage evaporates from the body in the form of perspiration.

Ideal Diet

There is no one ideal diet because every individual is different and needs differ. Basically we could live and be quite fit by living entirely on milk, wholemeal bread, and green vegetables, but it would be a very boring diet. A daily average diet can include a certain amount of milk and cheese, bread and cereals, meat, and fresh fruit and vegetables – that would certainly cover your basic requirements, but remember the old maxim: enough is as good as a feast. The greatest danger in our society today is eating too much, so it is important to select the right diet for you – and stick to it.

Chapter Seven

Selecting the Right Diet and Sticking To It

To be certain that you are receiving good nutrition, keeping fit and healthy, and at the same time remaining basically the correct weight for your build, you have to choose the right diet for YOU. This need not mean a vast change in your present diet or lifestyle, but just a little more thought and careful planning. A case of 'think before you eat'. But never forget that eating should be a pleasure. It is one of the joys of life to sit down and enjoy a good meal, so in your effort to keep fit don't make the mistake of thinking of food only in terms of nutrients, vitamins, carbohydrates and calories, otherwise eating will become a chore and a bore. If you do not enjoy your food then your mental attitude towards eating is wrong, and obviously if you don't find it relaxing and you consider cooking a strain then it will have some bearing on your general outlook and health.

Cooking can in fact be very therapeutic and a satisfying skill. My wife happens to be a great cook and I thoroughly enjoy my meals. She is Italian so we do eat a lot of Italian food, although we avoid anything too fattening. Fortunately I've got a very high metabolism so I can eat pastas without putting on weight. The important thing in cooking is to have a varied diet where possible, and if you try new recipes frequently, at least one new dish a week, you will find that mealtimes become an adventure. It need not be time consuming either if you plan carefully. Involve the whole family in the preparation so that it becomes something you have created together. It need not be a case of 'too many cooks' if you each have your own task to perform, and you will find that kids are far less fussy if they have actually helped prepare the meal themselves.

When dealing with the family it is important to avoid telling them how nutritious the dinner is, and how much fitter they will be, because this will tend to put them off. Just let them enjoy it for what it is. You will have the satisfaction of knowing they will be fitter! They'll soon notice the difference too when they start eating fresh food instead of pre-packed convenience foods.

Good health and good eating need not be expensive or time consuming if you just take a little extra care. For example, when buying meat try and buy leaner cuts that have less fat on them, and buy a little less meat and a little more vegetable instead. Your plate and stomach will be just as full, and yet it will be a much healthier meal. If you buy fresh or frozen vegetables, don't overcook them as this will destroy the vitamin content. Eat as much of the vegetable as you can: even carrot tops can be cooked.

Think carefully about your methods of cooking too. You may be cooking food wrongly, making it more fattening than it need be and spoiling the taste too. For instance, steamed vegetables retain their full taste and their vitamin content, much more than boiled vegetables. Where possible, grill food rather than fry it, and if you do have to fry, then get the fat really hot before putting in the food, this way less will be absorbed. Pressure cookers are ideal for cooking meats and vegetables and in half the time too. Try experimenting with meats – many delicious dishes can be made from inexpensive chicken livers and other offal. There are also many varieties of fish available now, and a dish, such as kedgeree, made from fish and eggs, is a complete meal in itself and of great nutritional value.

Salad stuffs are available throughout the year, so try and eat a salad at least once a week, and vary it by adding chopped raw vegetables, vegetable tops, raw mushrooms, nuts, fruit, peppers, and the like. Replace puddings and sweet desserts with fresh fruit where possible, again you don't have to stick to the same boring fruits, but experiment with new varieties of fruit that are available at your market.

On the whole, the best advice anyone can give regarding your diet is not to worry too much about it. Eat sensibly and wisely, not to excess and indulging in food that you know is bad for you, especially if you happen to be overweight. Choose a diet that is satisfactory to your bodily requirements, your lifestyle, and your pocket. Make eating something that you will enjoy, and remember that there are other things in life which are just as important, so don't make it the be-all-and-end-all of your day. The following guidelines should help you choose your daily diet, depending upon your basic build.

Eating to Stay Slim:

We have already looked at the problem of being overweight, and know that it is caused by an excess of calories, which are stored as fat. There are many causes of obesity, it could be that you have a low metabolism, perhaps it is hereditary or you were overfed as a child, or maybe you are just downright greedy! Whatever the cause, if you do happen to fall into the 'overweight' category, it is most important that you pay particular attention to your diet. This does not mean that you have to starve or live entirely on water and lettuce, but it does mean that you have to choose your food more carefully and rethink your lifestyle.

Many people eat far more than they really need out of boredom; they eat between meals, whilst at the theatre or watching TV, and having got overweight they lack the willpower to do anything about it.

The Health Education Council have devised a method of staying slim, without having to continually count calories, and by following their advice you can keep in shape and feel great at the same time. It is called the 'Traffic Light Guide', in which food is divided into three groups according to their calorie concentration. Use the three groups to discover a sensible balance which suits you.

The Traffic Light Guide:

Red (High in calories) – Stop and think . . . Sugar, sweets, chocolate, cakes, pies, pastries, biscuits, heavy puddings, honey, syrup, treacle, jam, marmalade, fruit tinned in syrup, dried fruit, cream, butter, margarine, lard, cooking oil, fat on meat, salad dressing, salad cream or mayonnaise, chips, crisps, peanuts, aperitifs, spirits and liqueurs, most soft drinks and mixers.

Amber (Medium in calories) – go carefully . . . Fatty meats (like bacon or salami), sausages, liver pate, eggs, milk, oily fish (like herring, mackerel, sardines, tuna, salmon), cheese (except cottage cheese), thick creamy soups, nuts, bread (eat wholemeal or brown rather than white), cereals, rice, pasta (like spaghetti and macaroni), potatoes, savouries. Ready made-up dishes. Wines, beers and cider.

Green (Low in calories) – go right ahead . . . Fresh fruit, salads, green and root vegetables, white fish, seafood, poultry, game, kidney, heart, brain, cottage cheese, yoghurt (natural), skimmed milk, bran, consomme and clear soups, herbs and spices, low-calorie soft drinks, coffee and tea (without milk), saccharine, water.

If, as you eat, you choose food carefully from each category, remembering to eat only very little from the RED-group through to as much as you like from the GREEN-group, you will remain slim and healthy. It is far easier to stay slim than it is to lose weight, so a little care choosing what you eat and enough regular exercise will go a long way to get you feeling really great.

If, however, you are overweight and for you it is not a case of staying slim, but a matter of losing a few pounds, then make up your mind to lose the excess by increased exercise and a reducing diet.

Losing Weight

To become slim when you are overweight is a matter of watching very carefully *all* that you eat. Unfortunately there is no secret formula, and no medicines, potions or pills will help you shed those excess pounds. The answer is to make yourself determined to lose weight at all costs. A will to succeed is half the battle.

There are many slimming diets available and it is important to choose one that is going to suit you. If you are really overweight, and it's not just a result of over-indulgence at Christmas, then your doctor will give you a diet sheet to help you plan your meals. If you are going to slim, look closely at your eating habits. Do you eat because you are hungry or is it purely habit that you eat four cream-crackers and ¼lb cheese each evening while watching the news? Do you unconsciously pick up food whilst watching TV without even realising it?

To diet seriously you must start TODAY. Don't wait until tomorrow because you know tomorrow never comes. Weigh yourself now, and if possible get yourself a little exercise book and start a new page every day. Write your weight at the top of the first page, the day you begin your diet, and if, for example, it is a Tuesday, weigh yourself every Tuesday at the same time and write it down so that you can see week by week how much you have lost.

At the end of each day write down exactly what you have eaten, don't forget all those cups of tea and coffee, and add up your daily calorie intake. You will find that this acts as an incentive because you will feel very cross with yourself if you see that one day's calorie total was far in excess of the previous day, and you will find yourself trying to beat a certain target. A fun way to slim is to diet with your friends. Check each other's daily calories. Be honest and don't forget to write down those biscuits you had mid-morning and that chocolate whilst watching the late-night horror film, because the only one you are cheating is yourself.

Help yourself whilst slimming by not buying tempting food, such as chocolate biscuits. If you haven't got it in the house you can't be tempted to eat it! Always make your food look appetising and make it varied. Use a smaller plate too, that way you can eat less without realising it. You will also get slim much quicker if you start taking some regular exercise, as this will burn up any excess calories, and will also help you sleep better, and will take your mind off food!

Set yourself a daily calorie allowance. The average man needs between 2,500-3,000 calories a day, the average woman between 2,000-2,500. If you have less calories then your body will make up for it by using up the excess weight stored in the body. If you only have 1,500 calories a day your body will compensate by using roughly one pound of fat a week – and you will get slim!

Don't go completely mad and cut down too much, as that will only make you ill and you could be lacking in vitamins, so eat food that has high nutritional value such as green vegetables, fish, liver, low-fat cheese, chicken and low-fat meats, and try and eat some bran daily too.

As a general rule, don't eat less that 1,500 calories a day. If you find that one day you have had an extremely low calorie intake, say less than 1,000, then make up for it the next day by eating a little more. Some people like to keep their calorie intake very low during the week, so that they can eat more at weekends; this is fine as long as you are sensible, and it may make your dieting much easier for you, especially if you are at home with the family at weekends and haven't the will-power to watch them eating!

Success, as in all things, will come only through perseverance and the will to succeed. Try and avoid alcohol, as this is fattening. If you must nibble between meals or whilst watching TV then eat fruit or raw vegetables which will be much more satisfying.

There are many pamphlets and books available which will give you the calorie content of most foods. Some are really comprehensive and give you particular brand products, and as much detail as the difference between the calorific value of an apple whether green or red, cooked or raw. Here, however, is a basic guide to calorific values, so begin now and see how many calories you've eaten so far today already.

Calorific Values

		PER OUNCE	AMOUNT	CALORIES
Dairy Produce & Fats				
Cheese	Cheddar	88	Average helping	100
	Dutch	103	Average helping	100
	Cream	232	1 tablespoon	150
Cream	double	132	1 tablespoon	80
	single	62	1 tablespoon	38
Eggs	raw or boiled	46	1 egg	80
	omelette	57	2 eggs	200
	scrambled	79	1 tablespoon	250
	poached	45	1 egg	80
	poached & toast	130	2 eggs & 1 piece of toast	300
	fried	68	1 egg	140
Lard		262	1 tablespoon	180
Butter		226	2 small pats	100
Margarine		226	2 small pats	100
Milk	fresh	19	1 pint	380
	condensed or evaporated	100	1 tablespoon	80
	fresh, in tea	80		10
Yoghourt	natural	15	4 oz pot	60
	fruit flavours	27	4 oz pot	108
Meat, Poultry & Game				
Bacon	back, fried	169	3 rashers	340
	gammon	126	1 thick rasher	380
	streaky	149	3 rashers	350
Beef	corned	66	3 slices	150
	roast sirloin	109	4 slices	330
	steak, grilled	78	1 medium	320
	steak, fried	86	1 medium	350
	steak, pudding	68	3 tablespoons	350
	steak, stewed	31	3 tablespoons	175
Beefburghers	fried	75	2	150

		PER OUNCE	AMOUNT	CALORIES
Bolognese sauce		39	3 tablespoons	244
Chicken	roast	29	4 slices	150
Curry	meat	48	3 tablespoons	300
Ham		123	3 slices	250
Irish stew		39	3 tablespoons	350
Lamb	chop, fried	146	1 medium	300
	chop, grilled	108	1 medium	250
	leg, roast	83	4 slices	250
Liver	fried	74	2 medium slices	280
Pork	chop, fried	128	1 medium	400
	leg, roast	90	4 slices	300
Rabbit	stewed	26	3 tablespoons	100
Sausages	beef	81	2 large	250
	pork	93	2 large	280
Shepherds pie		34		
Steak & kidney pie		85	3 tablespoons	400
Turkey		34	4 slices	170

Fish

		PER OUNCE	AMOUNT	CALORIES
Cod	steamed	19	medium steak	110
	fried	39	medium steak	200
	grilled	36	medium steak	180
Fishfingers	fried	57	3 fishfingers	171
Haddock	steamed	21	1 medium fillet	84
Herring	baked	50	1 medium fish	250
	fried	59	1 medium fish	300
Kipper		31	Medium pair	200
Plaice	steamed	14	1 medium	100
	fried	40	1 medium	200
Pilchards		2	6	40
Salmon	fresh	46	1 medium steak	180
	tinned	39	2 tablespoons	140

Vegetables

(Most vegetables have a low calorific value. For example, Runner Beans 2 per oz.; Sprouts 5; Courgettes 2; Lettuce 3; Onions 4; Carrots 5; Mushrooms 2; Cauliflower 3; etc. This is if boiled, steamed, or raw. Onions, for example, are 4 calories boiled, but 101 calories fried!)

		PER OUNCE	AMOUNT	CALORIES
Beans	Baked	27	On 1 slice toast	180
	Broad	12	2 tablespoons	50

		PER OUNCE	AMOUNT	CALORIES
Beans	Butter	26	2 tablespoons	80
Beetroot	boiled	13	3 slices	30
Corn	boiled	25	2 tablespoons	100
Lentils	boiled	27	2 tablespoons	80
Parsnips	boiled	16	3 tablespoons	50
Peas	fresh	14	3 tablespoons	60
	tinned	24	3 tablespoons	80
Potatoes	boiled	23	2 small	100
	baked	24	1 medium	80
	chips	68	2 tablespoons	300
	mashed	34	1 tablespoon	100
	new boiled	21	3 or 4 small	90
	roast	35	2 small	140

Fruits & Nuts

Apples	eating	10	1 medium	30
	cooking (baked)	9	1 medium	100
	cooking (stewed)	20	3 tablespoons	120
Bananas		22	1 medium	50
Chestnuts		49	4 nuts	30
Cob nuts		113	10 nuts	60
Dates		61	6 dates	130
Grapes		17	12 grapes	34
Grapefruit	fresh	3	1 medium	20
	tinned	15	3 tablespoons	60
Oranges		8	1 medium	40
Pears	eating	8	1 medium	32
Strawberries	fresh	7	6 large	20

Miscellaneous foods & cereals

Biscuits	cracker	158	2 biscuits	70
	digestive	137	2 biscuits	130
	sweet	158	2 biscuits	120
	water	126	2 biscuits	110
Bread	white or brown	69	1 slice	80
Cornflakes		104	6 tablespoons	100
Doughnuts		101	1 medium	250
Flour		99	1 tablespoon	70
Jam tarts		112	2 medium	300
Mince pies		111	2 medium	300
Oatmeal porridge		13	3 tablespoons	80
Rice		35	2 tablespoons	130

	PER OUNCE	AMOUNT	CALORIES
Ryvita etc	110	2 pieces	50
Sandwiches savoury		1 round	300
Shortbread	148	1 piece	120
Yorkshire pudding	62	1 slice	70

Drinks

	CALORIES	
Coffee – black	0	
white	30	
Tea – with lemon	0	
with milk	25	
Drinking chocolate	250	
Champagne – dry	90	
sweet	120	
Brandy – 1 measure	75	
Cola drinks – 1 glass	90	
Low calorie drinks	1	
Dry ginger	24	
Gin – 1 measure	70	
Vodka – 1 measure	90	
Sherry	100	
Port	135	
Tonic water	36	
Soda water	0	
Lager – 1 pint	165	
Bitter – 1 pint	182	
Cider (sweet) – ½ pint	119	
White wine (dry) – large glass	75	
White wine (sweet) – large glass	107	
Red wine – large glass	75	

If you do have sugar. Remember it is 25 calories per teaspoonful! So black coffee is 0 calories, but add two sugars and it's 50 calories!

You will see that alcohol is very high in calories so should be avoided if at all possible. Drink low calorie drinks. If in a social atmosphere you don't want to feel conspicuous with a glass of orange juice – have a glass of tonic or soda water, no one will realise that it's not a double gin and tonic!

A careful check on your calorie intake will help you maintain the required level to keep you slim. No one can pretend that slimming is easy, because it isn't, it takes willpower. But when you consider what excess fat does to you, you cannot help realising how worthwhile it all is. A final frightening fact is that every ten pounds of fat in your body requires *six miles* of minute blood vessels to maintain it! That is putting a tremendous strain on your heart, and your health in general, so get rid of it now!

Checking Your Weight

Obviously there really is no average weight because everyone is different in build, bone structure, and so on. You will find that nearly every book on general fitness will give you a guide to what your correct weight should be depending upon your height. I weigh fifteen stone so should probably be 7' 2" tall! Below is a table of heights and weights of the average person, but as no two people are alike, the average person does not exist, so only use the chart as a very basic guide.

WEIGHT (in ordinary indoor clothing, in pounds)

HEIGHT	MEN	WOMEN
5' 1"	129	120
5' 2"	133	123
5' 3"	136	126
5' 4"	139	129
5' 5"	143	133
5' 6"	147	137
5' 7"	152	141
5' 8"	156	145
5' 9"	160	150
5' 10"	165	154
5' 11"	170	158
6' 0"	175	162
6' 1"	180	167
6' 2"	185	171

Guides to Losing Weight

There are many diets available so you must choose one to suit you, your tastes and lifestyle. Whilst dieting try and get a balance between plenty of exercise and plenty of rest too so that you don't feel exhausted. Never starve yourself completely as this can be dangerous. It is much better to cut down gradually on your food and get into the habit of eating less. Drink plenty of liquid too, at least three glasses of water a day. It is always unwise to cut down on liquid, however much less food you are eating. Avoid crash diets too, these can so easily lead to anorexia nervosa without you even realising it. Don't be fooled into thinking that a certain food will help you to slim either, for example many people think that eating grapefruit will break down your fat, it won't. It is a good fruit to eat when slimming as it is high in vitamins and low in carbohydrates, but it will not in itself help you slim. There is nothing that is going to beat a simple reduction in food and a sensible well planned diet, plus the necessary determination to succeed.

How to Put on Weight

Yes, believe it or not, there are people who *need* to put on weight; not everyone comes under the heading of 'fatties'. This problem can often be just as distressing and as difficult as trying to lose weight. We live today in a society where it is fashionable and desirable to be slim, it means you can wear what you like, eat what you like, and generally means you are much fitter and more agile too.

But there are people who are underweight, perhaps because they have suffered a serious illness and need building up, or because they have a very high metabolism and use a lot of energy. Maybe they are just naturally skinny and generations of their family have been bean-poles. It is often the case too that people who are painfully thin do not really find eating a pleasure, they eat because it is essential to life, but it is a part of life that they take for granted and never look forward to.

If you are thin and want to put on weight, or have tried but found however much you eat you still stay the same, then you too have to plan your diet carefully, and, like the slimmers, start today. Get yourself an exercise book and divide it into days, as explained earlier, and write your present weight at the top of the first page, weighing yourself weekly thereafter to see how much you have gained.

Now have a serious think about WHY you are thin. Do you worry a lot about things? If so, make a conscientious effort to relax more. Do you miss out on meals altogether, and are you totally indifferent to food?

Make sure that you have one good meal every day, and for the first few weeks make sure you eat things that you will really enjoy. Don't make the mistake of giving yourself large platefuls either, this will only make you feel sick. Instead, increase your daily intake gradually, put on one extra potato and an extra slice of meat. Have a glass of wine with your meal too. Drink plenty of milk, replace your mid-morning coffee with a glass of milk and a biscuit or two, or make your hot drinks with boiled milk.

Don't neglect exercise either, as building up your muscles will keep you fit and make you look more substantial. Regular exercise, even if only a brisk walk, will help your appetite so you will eat more. Be sensible about your diet, never sit and eat a whole box of chocolates in the vain hope of putting on weight, you must put on weight gradually, just as a slimmer must take it off gradually. Eat plenty of dairy products and carbohydrates, such as potatoes, bread, and pastries, eat tinned fruits in syrups, and try experimenting with new and tasty dishes so that you begin to find food exciting. If you enjoy foreign food then eat pasta and rice, or if you like plain English food then there's nothing like good old Yorkshire pudding and pancakes to help you put on weight.

As with all diets it is a case of a sensible and healthy attitude towards your diet, regular meals, sufficient sleep, and a desire to succeed. If you have suddenly become thin for no reason then it would be wise to visit your doctor just to check that there is nothing physically wrong. If you are just naturally slim, then don't worry about it – you are someone to be envied by many. Take heart in the fact that slim people are often much healthier, suffer fewer illnesses, and live longer too!

Good health diets

Having considered both the 'fatties' and 'skinnies' of our population, we must not forget that a high percentage of people are not over or under weight and are really quite happy as they are. However it is just as important for them to be sensible about their eating habits. Just because you are the correct weight for your build does not mean you do not have to bother with a healthy diet.

Many people find that they are allergic to a certain food substance; eggs may cause a rash, spicy food may give you heartburn, and such people will know from their own experience which foods they should avoid, but occasionally you find people who have a specific medical complaint who still eat dishes that aggravate their condition. People with a condition called diverticulitis (a small pocket in the bowel), are told by the doctor not to eat peas – yet many still indulge occasionally even though they know that they will suffer afterwards.

Millions suffer from arthritis, and this can be linked to certain foods. Medical research has not yet brought any conclusive evidence, but tests in America have shown that arthritic conditions may be improved when patients eat plenty of fish and seafood, vegetables and rice. Dairy products, meat and chocolate had an adverse effect and so should be avoided.

Whatever your general state of health, a sensible diet is necessary to long life. Avoid sugar, fatty meats, and alcoholic substances, eat plenty of fruit, fresh vegetables, skimmed milk, wholegrain breads, white or lean meat. If your philosophy is 'all things in moderation' you shouldn't go far wrong.

Some people avoid meat altogether and become vegetarians, which is generally thought to be healthier and cheaper, and involves less chemical processing and cooking. However, if you just cut out meat and still eat white bread, tons of sugar and syrups, and overcook your vegetables, you will soon find your health far worse than if you had stuck to meat. To get all the required nutrients, the vegetarian must eat plenty of grains and pulses, dairy products, fresh fruit and vegetables, nuts, eggs and cheese to replace the proteins and amino acids that meat would have supplied. So before embarking on vegetarianism, remember that it is more than just cutting out meat from your diet, it is a whole new way of life. You must look into the subject very carefully before embarking on a meatless life, otherwise you could seriously damage your health.

So, you see, we really are what we eat. A good, natural healthy diet will keep you fit, healthy and in perfect condition. A haphazard and lax diet will leave you open to all kinds of physical disorders. Even if you feel fit now you may feel the adverse results of poor diet later in life when it is too late. Look after your body now, and it will look after you for as long as you want it to.

Chapter Eight

Sensible Attitudes to Drinking and Smoking

Your Life up in Smoke

If you are one of the many smokers in Britain, whether you smoke one cigar a week or fifty cigarettes a day, you'll probably try and skip this section of the book, pretending the pages got stuck together. You've heard it so many times before; you *know* smoking is bad for you. 'But', you might say, 'Grandad smoked until he was eighty-four and never got lung cancer. I know hundreds of people who smoke and seem to be alright. OK, some people die horribly painful deaths as a result of smoking, but why should that happen to me?'

Before you take another puff of that cigarette, perhaps you would like to know not what *might* happen to you, but what *will* happen to you if you carry on. You might just as well roll up your own death-warrant and smoke that instead . . .

Smoking gives people a feeling of security; it is comforting, like a dummy is to a baby. The only difference is that tobacco smoke contains over 300 different chemicals which enter your lungs and form a thick brown tar. If you smoke, for example fifteen cigarettes a day for nearly two years, that is 10,000 cigarettes and nearly half a pound of tar in your lungs. If you've been smoking fifty a day for twenty years . . . the mere thought is horrifying! That tar contains substances that induce cancer. They don't actually cause it, but there is actual proof that smoking accelerates cancer. Nicotine itself is a poison which in time affects the nervous system and, even if you don't inhale, 10% will still be absorbed into the body.

Smoking will slowly damage your lungs by breaking up the cells as the dirt and tar collects in them. Smoke also reduces the amount of air that reaches the lungs and blocks up the bronchial tubes. Phlegm builds up in the lungs causing a smoker's cough and, eventually, bronchitis due to the bacteria that are in the lungs of smokers. Bronchitis can easily become chronic resulting in death.

Cancer is triggered off as the smoke contains 'carcinogens' which promote cancer, thus making smokers seventy times more susceptible to lung cancer than nonsmokers. It is not only cancer of the lungs that can occur either, but in the mouth, throat, oesophagus, bladder, stomach, and larynx.

Because you breathe in the smoke and so less oxygen, naturally the carbon monoxide in cigarette smoke gets into the bloodstream, and so into every organ of the body. This puts a tremendous strain on the heart, causing thrombosis and blood clots.

One of the greatest risks is to pregnant women who smoke. It not only raises the risk of miscarriages and stillborn babies, but can seriously damage the health of the unborn baby in the womb, and tests prove that babies of mothers who smoked during pregnancy are much lighter in weight.

This is just a little of the medical evidence of what happens to the bodies of people who smoke. If you value your life and your health, why put yourself at risk? Two out of five smokers die before they are sixty-five, many don't even reach forty. So how can you live a longer life when you are reducing your life expectancy daily? Pipe and cigar smoking is dangerous, cigarette smoking is fatal.

Unfortunately it is not only your own health you are risking, but the health of your family and friends too. If parents smoke, their children run a much greater risk of catching colds and bronchitis, and other lung ailments. Your non-smoking friends will get minor eye irritations, headaches, and lung infections from *your* cigarette, just by breathing in what you exhale and having to be in the same smoky atmosphere.

Are you beginning to get the message? All right, smoking relaxes you, you enjoy it, it is a socially acceptable habit, it gives you something to do when you are bored. *But* you will already have discovered it is habit forming – you can't stop. It makes your clothes smell, your breath smell unpleasant, it stains your fingers, rots your teeth, affects your sex life, causes an early menopause in women, causes wrinkles around your eyes, reduces your senses of smell and taste, and it is very expensive, not only to your own pocket, but to the country as a whole. 20% of the total loss of working days is caused by illnesses related to smoking, many of them due to accidents. Smokers are far more prone to accidents than non-smokers because smoking slows down the reflexes. Don't you think it's about time you stopped smoking?

Cigarettes are drugs, once you are addicted it is not easy to stop. Yes, you *want* to stop, but how? You know that you will suffer from withdrawal symptoms, be irritable and bad tempered, depressed, but that will pass, and in fact breaking the habit might not be as difficult as you think if you go about it in the right manner.

How to stop smoking

Over eight million people in Britain alone have already successfully stopped smoking. Every week hundreds more kick the habit. What's their secret? How have they managed? Is there some miracle cure?

Sadly no. There's no foolproof formula for giving up smoking. No easy way. You might as well face the fact that giving up smoking is going to be a bit of a battle. But it's a battle you can win if you apply a little psychology. No one else can win this battle, only you. You must take complete command, but what a victory it will be in the end!

Firstly, you must make up your mind that you are definitely going to give up smoking. A half-hearted attempt is doomed to failure. Unless your willpower is turned full on, the habit will soon get a grip again. You've got to really want to give up and make up your mind that you're going to. You've got to say to yourself: 'Right, this is really it, I'm stopping smoking.' And mean it. When you've done that you're more than half way to winning. So, to help you with the big decision, here's a reminder of the very good reasons why eight million people have already made it.

* Just remind yourself that a cigarette smoker, on average, shortens his life by *five and a half minutes* for each cigarette smoked – not much less than the time spent smoking it.

* Just remind yourself that cigarette smoking causes the premature death of more than 50,000 people in this country *every year*.

* Just remind yourself that the average smoker has *double* the risk of dying from heart disease.

* Just remind yourself that the average smoker is several times more likely to develop chronic bronchitis – a progressive, crippling lung disease.

* Just remind yourself that smokers – even cigar and pipe smokers – are up to ten times more likely to get cancer of the mouth or throat.

* Just remind yourself that cigarette smokers, depending on how many and for how long they smoke, increase their risk of lung cancer by up to *twenty-five* times.

* Remind yourself what smoking is doing to you *now* – the cough, the shortness of breath, the awful taste in the morning, the constant colds and sore throats.

Are you playing Russian roulette with someone else's life?

Positive thinking. The very moment you stop smoking you start living longer, you will start living better, and will be fit for life. Your heart and lungs will work more efficiently and your blood will carry more oxygen. You will be less wheezy and puffed whenever you exert yourself. You'll have more stamina and more staying power. You will be less susceptible to coughs and colds and your resistance to many illnesses will improve.

Not only that, you will look better, smell better and find better ways of spending the money. No more nicotine stains on your hands and teeth. You will suddenly begin to taste more subtle flavours in your food and appreciate the aromas around you. You will become a nicer, more relaxed person, and with all the money you've saved you can enjoy a fortnight's holiday in the sun. So begin your Plan of Action now . . .

Plan of Action. This plan has been designed by a psychologist and will lead you through every step of the process, from the moment you decide to stop smoking to the moment you realise you no longer want to smoke. Through this period, don't worry about the next day, or week, or month, or about how on earth you are going to manage without cigarettes. With the help of this plan, just take each day as it comes, one day at a time.

First, prepare yourself for the battle!

1 Get yourself a pen, an exercise book, and a money box.
2 On the first page of the book, list the reasons *why* you want to stop smoking. List them one by one, beginning with those that mean the most to you, and underline the really important points. You'll be using these notes later.
3 Tomorrow, or the next typical working day, every time you light up, make a note of the time, what you were doing (for example, reading, drinking coffee, taking a break, working, watching TV, etc.), and do this for every single cigarette during the whole day. The effort will be worth it in order to plan your tactics later on. Make yourself a twenty-four-hour Smoking Chart, like this:

NUMBER	TIME	WHAT WERE YOU DOING?
1		
2		
3		

and so on, depending upon the number of cigarettes

4 The day after you have filled in your smoking chart, check it through and sort out which cigarettes you smoked when you didn't really *need* to. Try to cut out these cigarettes today, but don't worry about the others for now.

5 Also today, and every other day from now on until you stop smoking altogether, keep a tally of the cigarettes you smoke using a Daily Record chart. Just head your page morning, afternoon and evening, and put a little mark under the appropriate heading for each cigarette you smoke – and add them up at the end of the day.

6 All this chart-filling gives you a lot of useful information. You'll know how many you smoke, what time of day, which you need most or least, and how much your smoking varies from day to day.

7 When you've completed your daily record for a couple of days, it's time for you to fill in a Smoking Situation Chart. It's important because it will help you plan ahead. It consists of two columns:

When you most NEED a smoke	When you most ENJOY a smoke
1	
2	
3	

Here are some typical situations: answering the phone; listening to music; when bored; concentrating hard; having a drink with friends; taking a break; if alone; after a good meal, etc.

8 You are now ready to fix the day on which you stop. The idea is to stop smoking completely straight away. This is because research suggests that in the long run most people find it easier if they stop smoking suddenly and completely, rather than cut down gradually. The real secret is sheer determination and being prepared for difficulties. So pick the best day to stop.

If you smoke a lot at work, when you are tense or under pressure, then stop at the beginning of the weekend.

If you smoke more when you are relaxing or having fun, then stop on a Monday morning. Mark it in your diary and tell as many people as you can.

9 The evening before. Smoke your last cigarette and make sure you have none left. Either smoke them all or throw the rest away. It may help if your family and friends are witness to this historic act!

10 Now think about tomorrow – DAY ONE – the day you wake up a non-smoker, the first day of your new life.

Before you go to sleep, look at your list of 'Reasons for Stopping' and make up your mind to get through the day without a single cigarette. Check your 'Smoking Situations' chart and try to devise ways of avoiding them or counteracting them. It is mainly a matter of commonsense and determination. Read through what to do on DAY ONE and how you are going to cope with the difficulties. Now put out the light, and put smoking out of your life.

DAY ONE

1 This may be easier than you think!

At breakfast, read through your 'Reasons for Stopping' just to remind yourself why it is such an important decision; perhaps one of the most important of your life.

2 Read your 'Smoking Situations' chart. How are you going to cope with those difficult situations? Try to think up little ways to comfort or distract yourself. Some will work better than others. But you can get by, especially with a little help from your friends.

3 Here are some 'Helpful Hints' for difficult situations.

Mouth. Do you feel the need for something in your mouth? Try chewing gum or sucking a sweet (preferably low-calorie). Fresh fruit, a carrot or even a pencil will give you something to nibble.

Hands. Do you feel awkward without a cigarette in your hands? Play with something else: that pencil again, or a key ring, a coin, worry beads, anything.

Tension. Missing that calming cigarette? There are several things to try. First, when the craving comes, do deep breathing for a minute or two. Breathe all the way in. Hold it for a few seconds, then breathe all the way out. Really stretch your lungs. This is better if done by an open window or in the fresh air.

Another technique is muscle relaxation. This takes a little practice. All you need to do is sit comfortably with your eyes shut and then clench one fist as tight as you can.

Hold the tension for a few seconds and concentrate on it. Think what it feels like. Then release the tension *very* slowly. Keep releasing it for as long as possible. Feel the tension draining out of your hand. Now repeat the exercise with the other hand, then the arms, shoulders, neck and so on.

If you find you are very tense by the end of the day, try relaxing in a warm bath. If the tension is mainly in your neck and shoulders get someone to massage the muscles gently. Although a drink may help you relax, don't be too tempted to seek salvation in alcohol.

Habits. Does your daily routine seem odd without a cigarette? Then change it. Do everything you can to alter your activities so that you aren't constantly reminded of the need to smoke. For instance, if you used to smoke when you stopped for a cup of tea, try drinking something else instead: fresh orange juice, or hot soup, or simply less tea. It may help you to take your tea break at a different time or in a different place. Maybe go for a stroll.

Avoid situations where people are smoking. If possible, arrange things so that you work in the company of non-smokers. And try to spend more of your spare time with non-smokers. Always travel in no-smoking compartments or carriages. Remove all traces of smoking from your car. Make sure cigarette lighters and ashtrays are kept out of your sight whenever possible.

If you always smoked in the pub or club, you may have to steer clear of these danger spots over the next week or two. Don't worry, it won't be forever!

Relaxation. If relaxing was usually the time for a smoke, try keeping yourself occupied with a variety of chores or practical activities. Tackle some of those jobs that have been waiting to be done for ages, or take more exercise. Anything to keep your hands busy and your mind off smoking.

4   *Vitamin C* – Scientific research suggests that vitamin C may help to rid the body of nicotine. So from now on

drink plenty of fresh orange juice and/or eat lots of fresh fruit.

5 *Start saving* – Put 25p into the money box for each ten cigarettes per day you used to smoke. So if you smoked twenty a day, you'll collect a pound every other day. At current prices, someone who smoked twenty per day in five years would have saved over £1,000. You could certainly afford a nice treat for yourself as a reward for giving up! If you once smoked eighty a day you'd be saving yourself nearly £1,000 a year, and giving yourself a lot more years too by giving up.

6 DAY ONE SUMMARY – Take each day as it comes, and don't worry about tomorrow. Concentrate on getting through today, everyday. If you follow the plan it will be easier than you're expecting.

Day Two and Onwards

1 Each day look through your 'Reasons for Stopping' and check carefully the hints for Day One.
2 Find friends who also want to stop smoking. Persuade them to join you in making the break. You should, by now, be able to give them some good enough reasons for giving it up. You will find that you can give each other support and encouragement, and in a moment of weakness this could make all the difference between success and failure.
3 Try to develop new hobbies or interests that won't associate you with smoking. Spend less time at the pub or in front of the telly, and more time gardening, cooking, do-it-yourselfing, and join local classes or clubs. Try a new sport, badminton, squash, yoga, dancing. Become an action person.
4 Start each day in the right frame of mind, and if you are careful and determined, you will succeed.

Some Questions You Will Ask

1 Will it be difficult to stop smoking?
This depends how determined you are. Most people find

that once they really make up their minds to quit, it is surprisingly easy, despite some of the most obvious difficulties.

2 What difficulties?

The commonest problems are build-ups of tension, irritability, and difficulty in concentrating. You may feel awkward, uncomfortable and bored. This book gives you some helpful hints to overcome the problems, and good understanding support from family and friends will also help.

3 What causes these difficulties?

Just the loss of a habit which was very much part of your everyday life. It leaves a big gap and you are bound to miss it for a while. Although your body chemistry misses it too to some extent, you can't blame it all on nicotine or being 'addicted'. The main problem is simply changing a deeply ingrained habit.

4 How long will these difficulties last?

For most people the first three to four weeks are the worst and it gets easier after that. It may be quite easy all the time. Some people have difficulties that last a little longer, but they're usually over after six to eight weeks. However, you must always beware of the occasional temptation.

5 What must I look out for after the first month?

Don't get over confident. It'll take time before you feel completely like a non-smoker. Be especially careful about other people who will offer you cigarettes. Practise saying: 'No thanks, I don't smoke'.

6 How soon will my health improve?

As soon as you stop smoking. And it will go on getting better as long as you stay off.

7 Can a heavy smoker stop as easily as a light smoker?

If he is determined enough, yes. But don't use that as an excuse for waiting until you're a heavy smoker before you stop.

8 Will stopping smoking make me put on weight?

You may find that for the first few months you eat rather more than usual. This may be partly because your sense of taste improves, increasing your appetite, and partly because you may find it a comfort to have something in your mouth. If the extra food you eat contains a lot of calories, you're likely to put on a few pounds, but this effect is usually only temporary. The appetite readjusts itself and the weight returns to normal. Meanwhile, avoid high calorie food containing too much sugar or fat. Stick to fresh fruit, savouries or saccharine-flavoured sweet things.

9   What about smoking-withdrawal groups?

These are groups of smokers giving up under the guidance of a trained counsellor. The withdrawal plan is usually similar to the one described here, but there may be additional slides and films. Many people find that it helps to give up in the company of others going through the same experience. Unfortunately, there are still very few organised withdrawal groups throughout the country, but of course there's no reason why you shouldn't form your own informal group.

10   What about special tablets and filters to reduce the craving?

Some people find these helpful. The tablets either contain lobeline (a nicotine substitute) or something to make cigarettes taste awful. The filters work either by absorbing some of the nicotine (and tar) or by diluting it with air. Aids such as these may help you cut down your cigarette consumption but could also give you an excuse for continuing smoking rather than stopping altogether.

11   Will stopping produce immediate results?

Yes. Straightaway you'll feel fresher and smell fresher to your friends. The nicotine stains on your hands, teeth and hair will fade. Your tastebuds will come alive.

What's more, within hours, the efficiency of your lungs will improve. You'll find yourself less short of breath when you exert yourself, and you'll have longer staying power.

Within days the phlegm that has accumulated in your chest will start to loosen and over the next few weeks you'll cough it up. Already this will be reversing the progress of chronic bronchitis. At the same time your body and brain will adjust to the absence of nicotine in the bloodstream and the process leading to heart disease will switch into reverse.

The longer you stay off cigarettes, the more you cut your risk of lung cancer. You'll be fitter, stronger, and apart from all that . . . think of the money you'll be saving.

What Will You Have To Drink?

Drinking alcohol is part of the way of life for most people in this country. It is used not only as a drug to relieve the stress and tension of life, but it has also become a major social activity for many people. To have a pint in your hand is considered manly, and for many it is one of life's great pleasures. However, as everyone knows, drinking can have very unpleasant effects as well. When alcohol is consumed to excess, these effects can be serious and cause a considerable amount of harm. The task of everyone who wants good health is to learn how to enjoy alcohol sensibly, and without running the risk of harmful consequences to yourself and other people.

Social pressures often cause people to drink far more than they really want to. How many times has someone said 'Have one for the road before you go', and that drink might just be your last. That is why it is important not to pressurise people into having that last drink that they really don't want, or into having a hard drink when they really want a soft one. It is also important to respect those who choose not to drink at all.

Social pressures make it a lot harder to refuse a drink than to accept one. Drinking is made out to be masculine, sophisticated and tough. I tend to drink mainly wine, and only have a very occasional whisky for medicinal purposes, if I've got a cold or something, but that's all. I've seen what drink can do to people, and so have you, but it still takes a lot of courage to say 'No thanks', or 'Make my next one a tomato juice', because such a request makes those still drinking uneasy. If you do have the courage, however, you'll soon discover that people respect you for it, and may even follow your lead.

Learn How Much You Can Safely Drink. It is difficult to say exactly how much people can safely drink, because it varies from person to person, depending upon the mood, how much food has been eaten, energy level, and so on. Usually one or two drinks are not hazardous to anyone's health, unless you are grossly overweight, taking drugs, suffer from epilepsy or diseases of the liver, or have stomach ulcers.

There are a few important guides to follow whilst drinking, and if you follow these you should be OK.

1   Eat while you are drinking, even if it is only a packet of crisps. Alcohol is absorbed much more slowly into your bloodstream if you have food in your stomach, so you are less likely to get drunk. If you are going somewhere for a drink and know there won't be any food, then eat before you go.

2   There are many times that we drink when we aren't really thirsty. If you are tired or tense and you don't feel like a drink then don't allow yourself to be pressured into accepting one.

3   Avoid unfamiliar drinks, and especially mixing drinks. Drink slowly, don't gulp it down. Go for a while without a drink, or switch to soft drinks for a time. Beware of someone topping up your glass, it can lead you to drink far more than you realise.

4   NEVER drink to try and solve a problem. You could end up with two problems.

Drinking at Parties. Sometimes you may find yourself in a situation where heavy drinking is expected. This does not, however, mean that you've got to drink heavily. If you happen to be giving a party yourself then be sure to cater for people who don't drink at all, and remember that not everyone wants to drink alcohol all the time.

Provide plenty of food to accompany the drinks, and

encourage conversation so that drinking isn't the only attraction to the party. A few useful tips are:

* Don't fill glasses before they are empty.

* Don't rush to fill a glass if someone is drinking too fast.

* Decide when you want a party to end and close the bar an hour before this and serve coffee and snacks to give your guests the chance to wind down.

Drinking and Driving. I'm sure you've all seen someone who is hopelessly drunk and hopes no-one has noticed. But people do notice, and when you drink heavily it is often your family who suffer more than you do. We also know that drinking affects your driving, from the first drink onwards. Unfortunately, the more a driver has had to drink, the less able he is to detect this, as his judgement is impaired too. Tests with professional drivers have shown that they were unable to drive between moveable posts after a few drinks, and the more they drank the more certain they became that they could drive safely.

Over half the drivers involved in fatal accidents have alcohol in their bloodstream. Sobering up techniques, such as hot coffee, have no effect on alcohol that is already in your bloodstream. Only time does. If you are planning to drink, then make arrangements to be driven home, not only your licence is at risk, but your life.

How to treat people who have had too much to drink. Don't just ignore them, make sure they don't have any more drink. If you are the host then accept responsibility for their condition and look after them, offering them coffee, and give them somewhere to sleep until they are sober enough to go home safely, or arrange a taxi to take them home.

Whatever happens don't let them drive home, or you run the risk of being to blame for what happens.

A drinking problem. It is all too easy to let drinking become a problem. A few pints on their own may seem trivial enough, until one day the result is a serious accident for you

104

or someone else, at work or on the road. What starts out as light-hearted social drinking so often turns into a pattern of heavy drinking. This leads to a danger of becoming dependent on alcohol, and once that has happened it begins to turn into a very serious problem.

Social drinking can lead to alcoholism because the drinker finds it relieves stress, and he becomes increasingly more dependent upon drink. In early stages it leads to blackouts, feelings of guilt; he or she starts avoiding family and friends and refuses to discuss the problem, until eventually the body begins to deteriorate, behaviour becomes irrational, and eventually mental and physical deterioration lead to death. Alcoholism is a disease and must be treated as such. If you suspect someone in your family is becoming an alcoholic then get help for them immediately, either by visiting your doctor or Alcoholics Anonymous.

Here are some symptoms to look out for:
  * Drinking at irregular times, like in the morning
  * Skipping meals in order to drink
  * A preoccupation with drink, feeling it is a necessary part of life
  * Feeling guilty about drinking
  * A deterioration in reliability, and basic friendships.
  * Drink hidden and consumed secretly
  * Physical and mental deterioration, lack of sex drive, drop in working efficiency
  * Do other people comment on what is happening?
If you see any of these symptoms, then help is needed.

Constant alcohol consumption, even if it doesn't lead to alcoholism, will impair the digestion, resulting in vitamin deficiency, and cirrhosis of the liver, caused through alcoholic poisoning and nutritional neglect. Alcohol upsets the metabolism and slowly destroys the brain, and eventually every organ in the body (especially the kidneys and heart) will suffer.

The facts about alcohol. As with smoking, it is important that you understand the facts about drinking. Some drinks are obviously stronger than others (in terms of concentration of absolute alcohol) so you must choose your poison carefully!

The order of strength is:

Strongest: Spirits   40% alcohol
                Fortified wines e.g. sherry   20%
                Table wines   10%
Least: Beer   5%

Drinks are served in their various glasses and measures because obviously a pint of whisky would be much stronger than a pint of beer. The following measures are roughly equivalent:

½ pint beer = 1 glass of wine = 1 glass of sherry = 1 single whisky = 1 unit of alcohol

Most of the alcohol we drink is absorbed rapidly into the bloodstream through the walls of the stomach and intestine. The exact amount will depend upon how much you drink, and whether or not the stomach was empty, also the weight of the individual. For example, an eleven-stone man drinking one pint of beer: the amount of alcohol in his blood will rise until it reaches its peak after about one hour. It will take another two hours for the liver to 'burn' it all up.

We measure the amount of alcohol in your blood (always in milligrams) by seeing how much is in 100 millilitres of blood. So the eleven stone man, after drinking one pint, would have thirty milligrams of blood per 100 millilitres. A person weighing less would have a higher percentage.

The effect of alcohol. No-one can predict the effect accurately because people react differently depending upon their personality and how much they have drunk. Some people become boisterous, others sleepy. To some alcohol is a stimulant, to others a depressant. As soon as alcohol enters the bloodstream it effects judgement, self-control and skills.

Research proves that workers with blood levels between 30-100 mg have considerably more accidents than those below 30mg. Drivers with 30 mg (that's one pint of beer) are likely to have accidents. At 80 mg the likelihood is four times greater; at 150 mg it is TWENTY-FIVE times greater, that is after five pints of beer.

Here is the effect that drink will have:

NO OF DRINKS	BLOOD ALCOHOL LEVEL	EFFECTS
1 pint of beer	30 mg	Likelihood of having an accident begins to increase.
1½ pints beer or 3 whiskies	50 mg	One becomes cheerful. A feeling of warmth. Impairment of judgement and inhibition.
2½ pints of beer or 5 whiskies	80 mg	Loss of driving licence.
5 pints of beer or 10 whiskies	150 mg	Loss of self-control. E x u b e r a n c e. Quarrelsomeness. Slurred speech.
6 pints of beer or 13 whiskies	200 mg	Stagger. Double vision. Memory loss.
¾ bottle of spirits	400 mg	Oblivion. Sleepiness. Coma.
1 bottle of spirits	500 mg	Death possible.
	600 mg	Death certain.

What can that lunchtime drink do? Take, for example, a person who has a sherry, a couple of glasses of wine, and a brandy at a business lunch. This is five units of alcohol (if the brandy was a double) and a blood level of 75 mg. Although not above the legal limit, driving will still be affected.

If three hours later this person had a couple of pints of beer after work with friends, even before the first mouthful of beer, his blood level would still be at a raised level from lunch.

After just two pints the blood level would be above the legal limit because of the effects of lunchtime. He can now not only lose his driving licence, but is also over four times more likely to have an accident.

Side effects of alcohol. Alcohol contains calories, but really has no true nutritional value and so a regular intake of alcohol can easily lead to a problem of overweight, and the drinker's proverbial 'beer pot'.

Alcohol can cause aggressive and foolish behaviour, especially in the young. Many young girls find themselves in sexual trouble, and a major cause of death in young men is road accidents as a result of alcohol.

Experts agree that regular drinkers, (certainly those who drink several pints of beer daily), run a risk of social and health damage. Family problems; financial debts; violence in marriage; child neglect; separation and divorce.

Work problems; difficulties in personal relationships; poor work performance; lack of promotion and possible job loss.

Health problems; liver cirrhosis; heart disease; peptic ulcer; pneumonia; cancers of the digestive tract.

Even small amounts can sometimes be harmful, so stick to the following pattern:

* Respect alcohol – remember excessive amounts only lead to trouble.
* Always try and eat something while you drink.
* Drink slowly – never gulp.

* Do not drink alone.
* Resist the insistence that everyone must buy a round – to avoid appearing mean, offer to pay for something else.
* Always dilute spirits.
* Never drink when driving or using machinery.
* Never feel obliged to drink alcohol.
* Set a limit to the number of drinks you want and don't exceed it.

Remember. To enjoy life to the full it is not essential to drink. Drinking is not a sign of adulthood, sophistication, or toughness. Most people like a drink – but nobody likes a drunk!

Chapter Nine

Avoiding Stress and Strain

Stress is undeniably one of the increasing problems of modern life. We all suffer stress and strain at certain periods in our life, it is perfectly natural to us all. Basically it depends upon your temperament. I thank God that I've got an easy going temperament and it takes a lot to get me out of my stride. I don't get uptight, I don't want to fight and hit everyone. The biggest tension I used to have was about an hour before I went in the boxing ring. If I was away training for Muhammed Ali for five weeks in a training camp I never ever thought of him. I used to enjoy the training and then the day of the fight I'd think about who I was fighting, but I never got uptight.

Fortunately I had a good manager. You know that you've got all the friends and well-wishers in the world, but your manager knows that an hour before you're due in the ring is the most nerve-racking time of any fight so he clears the dressing room and keeps everyone out. Jimmy, my manager, used to let me be on my own because he knew that I didn't want to talk a lot. He would let me do just what I wanted to do, and I used to do deep breathing and relaxation exercises and everything would be fine.

Now that was my job, and it is often people's work that brings them the most pressures and therefore the most stress. People who have excessively demanding jobs, especially those with responsibility for other people's lives, may suffer from stress which can lead to anxiety, irritation, high blood pressure and stomach ulcers.

The average executive is also likely to suffer stress as a result of driving to work in the rush hour and getting to appointments on time. The occasional period of increased heart-rate will not do much harm, but for people whose jobs are either highly responsible, or dreadfully monotonous with no job satisfaction, there is an increased likelihood of illness caused by stress.

A third of our lives is spent working, and several hours may be spent each day travelling to work. It is obvious that there are more of us now than ever before – the population of the country has doubled in the last hundred years. Most of us have experienced being squashed into a rush-hour bus or train, and many people wonder if the sheer pressure of numbers is damaging our mental or physical health by causing stress.

When the body is stressed there are several physical signs. The heart rate rises, the skin goes pale, the digestion rate goes down and blood floods to the muscles. If stress continues we become irritable, there is loss of sleep and appetite, and full scale depression can set in. Heart diseases and stomach ulcers may be related to stress. Experiments with rats, show they become aggressive under stress and overcrowding, so environment is very important to our health.

Stress is nervous tension, and is not only caused by environment, but by psychological factors as well, such as financial worries or relationship problems. Environmental stress is caused by poor and perhaps noisy working conditions, or nearly being killed by a piece of machinery. Psychological stress is caused by unhappy home conditions, perhaps due to divorce or death, or unhappiness at work. All of this can cause intense feelings of frustration, and if this is prolonged and bottled up inside, it begins to cause physical as well as emotional tension, and can eventually become serious by making you physically ill.

If there is hostility or unhappiness at home, or perhaps feelings of intense loneliness, this can easily lead to stress. Likewise if work pressures are too great, or you don't like the job you are doing, it may become a great worry. Teenagers, especially, go through periods of great stress as they go through a period of self identification, encounter

111

relationship difficulties, and realise that they don't really know what they want from life. Growing up can be a hard and painful experience, but it is something we all go through and learn to cope with in the end.

How to cope with stress. If you feel tense and strained it is necessary to sit down and have a serious look at yourself. Try and sort out the problem and get things into perspective. The greatest step of all is realising that you have a problem and what it is. Once you can identify what is causing you stress, you can take steps to conquer it. In most cases the problem can be solved, and there is always an alternative to any situation if you really look for it.

We all react to stress in a different way, and a little stress now and again is healthy; too much can be fatal. Some people get their problems so out of perspective that their lives are constantly filled with stress and they would find it very hard to live a normal life.

Whatever is causing you stress remember that drink, drugs, or cigarettes are not the answer. In the long run they are a much bigger problem, their relaxing effect is temporary, their long term effect can be harmful to your health.

Don't try to avoid stress altogether either, but make use of it, and if you happen to be very tense then engage yourself in something energetic, such as sport, or even vigorous housework. The most important aspect of stress is to learn to relax. Relaxation and tension are antagonistic to each other, total opposites, and if you learn how to move from one to the other you will have the perfect balance in your life.

First, you must identify what is causing you stress, and once you know what it is you can take the first step to conquering it.

Identifying the causes. One of the major causes of stress, as we have already discovered, is work. Either the actual job itself, or the lack of work can both cause serious stress. If

112

you really hate your job, the people you work with, the unsociable hours, the paper work, then face up to the problem and attempt to change it. It is never too late to change your job, and if your present career is making you ill, then take immediate steps to change it. Obviously it is not an easy matter and may mean a large drop in salary and perhaps less security which your family might not appreciate, but it is far more important that you enjoy your career, it's no good making a lot of money if you are going to die of a coronary at fifty brought on by stress.

If after very careful thought you feel that a change of job is totally impractical then you have to get round the problem another way. The answer is to make your 'out of office' hours as enjoyable and fulfilling as possible. Take up new hobbies, begin evening classes, try a new sport, make new friends, this will give you lots to look forward to, and you may even find people at work have similar interests too and so open up totally new doors for you. If you've always hankered after being a writer or an artist, then try writing or painting in your spare time, you might eventually be able to sell your work, and who knows – your hobby may turn into a career.

Anyone who is out of work too should not just sit around and mope. Whether you're eighteen and can't get a job because you're too highly qualified but not enough experience (as is so often the case today), or middle-aged and made redundant, or even retired but young at heart, there is no reason why you should not make the most of your life. If you take up new hobbies, join societies, try some 'do-it-yourself' at home, you'll find it therapeutic, and hobbies will bring you into contact with people like yourself.

Life today is particularly distressing for the young, with threats of unemployment, and often a feeling of insecurity and an uncertainty as to which direction their lives should take. If you know young people who have problems, try and get them to talk about them. If it is career opportunities that are a worry then get them to visit a career counselling

113

service who will help them decide where to go. As I said earlier in the book, I'm a great believer in the philosophy that a 'kid's got to do what he wants', so don't try and push your children into jobs that they don't like, they will only be miserable and if things really don't work out, you will be the one that gets the blame.

Many problems stem from home life, often because husband and wife do not act as a partnership. Perhaps the husband has a demanding job and the wife feels neglected as a downtrodden housewife. Or maybe the wife goes out to work and the husband sees this as a threat to his masculinity and resents his wife working. As more women go out to work it is important to keep 'professional' and 'private' lives apart. If your general attitudes are right then there is no reason why home life should not be in perfect harmony.

Stress often occurs in both men and women over emotional conflicts and relationship problems. Living under the same roof with anyone, however much you love them, will obviously bring stress at times and a certain amount of tension. Quarrels and conflicts are part of human nature. Often there are communication problems between husbands and wives, parents and children, children and grandparents, but these could so easily be cured if people would only talk openly to each other. Tolerance is needed on all sides, and nothing helps relationships more than a frank and open discussion. So if there is a problem don't bottle things up inside you, clear the air and have a good old talk about it.

Finally, nearly everyone in their lives goes through some kind of personality problem that causes them stress. They may have a complex about something, perhaps a large nose, or a lack of self confidence. Or perhaps it is just part of their 'make-up' that makes them worry a great deal. For example, how stressed are you at the moment?

* Do you worry a lot about what other people think?
* Do you waste time worrying about lots of little things?

114

* Do you get easily irritated and cross?
* Do you feel tense and uncomfortable if someone asks you to do something for them?
* Do you worry about what people are saying about you?
* Do you find your heart beating very fast at times and your hands sweating?
* Do you find it difficult to sleep because so many thoughts are going through your head?

If the answer to any of these is 'yes', then you must learn how to overcome the stresses and strains of your everyday life. Here is what to do:

* Practise relaxation exercises as described in this book, especially deep breathing.
* Make sure you get plenty of daily exercise, it will help you sleep better too.
* If you get plenty of sleep, you will feel more refreshed and able to face each day. Your nerves will also be better.
* Make sure that your general health is good, that your diet is sensible and that you are not overweight.
* If you are a heavy smoker or drinker then try and cut down, or better still stop altogether.
* Whatever the situation try and remain calm, getting upset will *never* improve anything or gain anything, and will only make you much more tense.

Remember that life is for living, so try and enjoy it as much as possible. Everyone faces setbacks, has problems to face, and we know that it is all part of living, but nothing is ever worth making yourself ill. Whatever your problem, whatever is causing you stress, the most sensible thing you can do is *talk* to someone about it. It may be a cliché that a 'trouble shared is a trouble halved', but you'll find it's true.

Chapter Ten

Making the Most of the Breaks in the Day

Whatever your job or profession it is advisable to make the very most of your day, and maximise your time so that breaks are never wasted and become part of your daily fitness plan.

If you work in an office it is highly probable that you will spend much of your time sitting, and even though the mental work is exacting, it is physically undemanding. There are, however, measures you can take to make the most of your working situation to improve your health.

Before you begin work in the morning and when you finish in the evening, aim to make your travel to work as beneficial and enjoyable as possible. If possible, walk or jog to work as previously described. If you drive, you will probably have to put up with heavy traffic which will make you mentally and physically tense if you let it. So try instead to accept hold-ups from time to time and get into the habit of treating your drive as a pleasure. Always allow more than enough time for your journey so that you can relax.

Many people prefer or have to use public transport. Travel on trains or buses can build up tension just as much as driving. Here again, the key is to allow plenty of time. Avoid the smoking compartment if you have a chest or heart complaint. The air will certainly contain more carbon monoxide and other chest irritants than the air in a street full of traffic. If you must smoke on public transport always use the smoking compartment. Although you may get away with it you will certainly cause tension and resentment for other people. In fact for your own good avoid petty quarrels which so easily blow up in tense overcrowded situations.

Try and relax as much as possible on public transport,

although don't fall asleep and miss your stop! The rest will help you build up energy and cope with the rest of the day. If you let yourself get bad tempered, you'll simply arrive at work hot, flustered, and irritable for the rest of the day, which is not good for you or your colleagues.

Keep Fit at Work

Once at work, try and look after yourself as much as possible. For example, if your work is very detailed, be sure to take care of your eyesight. Have your eyes tested regularly, certainly every two or three years, but more frequently if you feel some deterioration.

If your optician says that you need glasses, then be sure to wear them – he knows what he is talking about. If the general lighting in your office is not adequate for your work, it is worth trying to get it improved rather than putting up with the glare of a desk lamp: frequent changes in the amount of light may strain your eyes and cause headaches. Do jobs like labelling equipment and files in such a way that you do not have to strain your eyes. During breaks try and splash your eyes with cold water, this will refresh them. Try to rest the eyes by closing your lids for a few minutes, or just by gazing into the distance. Your eyes are very valuable, so look after them.

The harder and more responsible your work is, the more essential it is for you to get enough rest during the day, and be sure to unwind completely at the end of it. Very few people seem able to relax completely, so it is necessary to learn how. Sit in a comfortable chair and take regular deep breaths. On breathing out relax one part of your body. It may be easiest to relax your toes first, then your knees, then your abdomen, then your fingers, the back of your neck, and lastly your eyebrows. Relaxation should be combined with gentle concentration of your mind on something as far removed from your work as possible.

Avoid becoming a workaholic. Sometimes you may have to work overtime or take some work home. This will do no harm as long as you cultivate the ability to forget about work when you finish. Lock a mental door on it and close your mind to any problems.

Teabreaks. Try and have a good breakfast before you start work, not just a coffee or a cigarette. That way you will not need a snack mid-morning. If you eat then, you will spoil your lunch. A poor lunch will lead to an afternoon snack, and so on. Eventually you will spoil your early evening meal and so have a late one. Then your sleep can suffer. So at tea breaks, just have a cup of tea and no snacks.

At lunchtime have a light meal including fruit and salad. If you must eat sandwiches, remember the calorie problem. Have one good meal each day, either at lunch or in the early evening. If you are going out and expect to have no time for a meal, have a proper lunch, but take some light exercise after it.

Fresh air. Never lose an opportunity to get outside during the day. Do not eat your lunch over your desk and then just sit about. Make a point of really exercising yourself during your lunch break, which means getting at least slightly out of breath. If you must have a full lunch take a steady stroll. If you just have sandwiches then eat them in a park, or nearby river, and have a good walk before returning to work, even if it is only around the shops. If you cannot take exercise at work during the day, then take it in the evening. Take up a sport, dig the garden, or take the dog out for a walk; you'll feel much better afterwards.

Creating energy when your resources are low. Sometimes people feel tired during the day. If you constantly feel tired then you need to look carefully at your diet and general fitness, but all of us feel down occasionally. It can be quite worrying when you feel tired half way through the day, or have had a tough day at the office and really don't feel like the evening out which you had planned.

Women, especially, get tired during the day when looking after energetic young children on top of all the daily shopping, housework, cooking and so on. Often there

118

is a specific cause, such as a low blood sugar level, or lack of iron, even a weight problem, and medical advice should be sought if there is a constant feeling of inertia. If, however, your resources just happen to be low on a particular day, there are ways of creating energy to buck yourself up.

Regular exercise will do much to raise the level of energy in the body because it will keep your heart and lungs healthy and your circulation going. Being on your feet all day long does not necessarily mean that you are getting enough exercise, and this could be the answer to your problem. Being inside all day and not getting enough exercise and fresh air will make you feel sluggish and tired.

Older people, or those who are in all day, get tired and fatigued even when they don't seem to have done anything very active. The tiredness comes from a feeling of boredom, it is psychological. In this case it is necessary for the person to stimulate their brain and take up some new hobby or interest.

After a hard day on your feet, legs often become swollen. Try and rest them whenever possible, preferably by lying down with your legs higher than your head. Remove shoes and stockings and walk around for a time in your bare feet to let them breathe, and plunge them momentarily into cold water to freshen them up. A change of shoes will often make tired and aching feet feel less tired, so take a second pair of shoes with you to the office if you can.

If, however, you have the correct diet, and, most important of all, get plenty of rest, you should have enough energy to see you through any day. If you have been ill and weak, and need building up again then pay particular attention to your diet. Try and drink plenty of milk and get as much fresh air and exercise as you can, you'll soon discover that your energy returns. If possible have twenty minutes or so set aside each afternoon when you can put your feet up and completely relax, until you feel back to normal health once more.

Chapter Eleven

Patterns of Sleep

One of the very best ways to keep fit is to sleep! Believe it or not, we each spend approximately one-third of our life asleep. Very little is known about it, but we do know that people die quicker from a lack of sleep than they do from a lack of food. Sufficient sleep makes you look and feel healthy, insufficient sleep causes exhaustion and disorientation.

How much we require varies from person to person. Although eight hours is usually thought to be the average some people need far less, others require much more. Everyone's sleeping pattern is different. Tests show that sleep may be a chemical process. Although it is a way of getting rest, that is not the sole purpose of sleep otherwise simply lying down would be enough.

As we get older the need for sleep is reduced. New born babies sleep for most of the day, and as they get older they stay awake longer during the day. Some older people only need two or three hours sleep a night. There is no uniform pattern, although it is generally thought that most of us actually require less sleep than we think we do. Most of us, however, find a constant sleeping pattern that suits us, and if you are happy with it, then there is no need to change. One of the worst things you can do is to worry about sleep; if you just relax at the end of the day your body will soon tell you when and how much sleep you need. If you feel constantly tired, you lack energy, your eyes are dull, your skin is in poor condition, that is your body's way of saying 'Get more sleep'.

We do know that whilst we are asleep energy is restored to the body, we totally relax so that if we are moved whilst asleep our bodies are totally limp. Some illnesses induce people to sleep and it certainly seems to have a healing process. The main reason, though, is that it is the only time the brain can really rest. Even though it does not switch off completely it does rest from its normal function of controlling the body. Research on sleep and keeping people awake showed that people prevented from sleeping gradually went mentally deranged, although people woken up after a short sleep showed little ill effect.

Most of us dream every night, even if we cannot remember in the morning what we dreamt. On average we dream for approximately two hours every night, but this varies from person to person and from night to night. Obviously conclusive and accurate tests are impossible. All we know is that we do dream, but why or how . . . that is a mystery to man, and we can only guess at the answer. Dreaming is clearly an essential and necessary part of sleep and a healthy sign. The psychologist, Freud, suggested that in our dreams we experienced our unconscious needs and desires, our hopes and our fears. Perhaps that is why in nightmares we experience happenings that we have always secretly dreaded, and this has been stored up in our subconscious.

As I said, not a great deal is known about sleep, though I know I enjoy mine! We do know, however, that there are two sleep patterns – 'Orthodox' and 'Paradoxical' sleep.

ORTHODOX SLEEP is the stage when your body begins to slow down. Your heart rate and breathing become much slower and rhythmical, the brain less active and the whole body metabolism slows down. All the tensions in the body disappear, although our muscles still move unconsciously. No-one stays completely still at night as the muscles would become stiff and seize up. In a light sleep we move between thirty and fifty times in one night, but the deeper the sleep the less we move. In this sleep the body begins to fight infection and any dead body cells are replaced, that is why if you are ill sleep is good for you and will make you well again.

PARADOXICAL SLEEP is known as REM (Rapid Eye Movements) and is the stage in our sleep when we dream. Orthodox sleep rests the body, and this rests the brain. There is very rapid movement behind the eyelids as we dream, the brain is very active.

We all need both kinds of sleep to keep us mentally and physically fit. If we did not have paradoxical sleep our mental and emotional health would suffer greatly. Our patterns of sleep vary each night – depending upon how tired we are, what we've eaten, how relaxed we are, the temperature of the body – but on average we begin with orthodox sleep, which gradually gets deeper for about an hour. The sleeper then falls into paradoxical sleep, which is light at first and then becomes heavier. In one night we alternate between both kinds of sleep. Although about 75% more time is spent in orthodox sleep, the length of time for each type will vary, with the periods of paradoxical sleep becoming longer as the night progresses. Our deepest sleep is the first long deep sleep (after we have been asleep about an hour) and after that sleep is much lighter.

If for any reason you lack paradoxical sleep (REM) for a few days, say for example you have a new born baby who wakes you up continually just as you are beginning to dream, the body will make up for it by changing your sleep pattern and you will begin to dream for very long periods, probably nightmares, until the body has regulated itself. One side effect of sleeping pills is that they stop REM sleep, so that when you stop taking them the body will make up for it. That is why sleeping pills tend to lose their effect after a while, and it is unwise to take them unless it is really necessary. A few sleepless nights of tossing and turning will not do you any real harm if you are fit and get plenty of exercise. All of us go through periods of sleeplessness if we have a worry, perhaps one of the family is ill, or we have an exam to take, but that is perfectly natural.

Some people, however, cannot sleep for medical reasons. Insomnia can be very unpleasant, but in fact the person may sleep without even realising it and so feel as if he has been awake all night. It can be caused by many reasons, perhaps a heart or lung disorder that will make breathing uncomfortable, but in many cases the problem is not medical at all.

Insomnia can occasionally be a result of tension or excitement, poor air conditioning, the bedroom too hot or too cold, bedclothing that is too light, intense pain, emotional upset or depression. It is often due to lack of exercise or bad food habits such as eating a heavy meal before going to bed.

On the opposite end of the scale we have somnambulism, or sleep walking, the name given to the condition when people may get up and walk around whilst still sleeping. This occurs when the part of the brain controlling your muscles stays awake, and so even though you are totally unconscious of what you are doing your senses are still partly awake and you move around the house with your eyes closed. This is often a frightening experience for other members of your household, but is quite harmless.

If you find difficulty in going to sleep at night, don't get into the habit of taking sleeping pills. These should only be taken during periods of great stress, such as the death of a loved one. Although there really is nothing worse than lying in the dark trying to get to sleep, the more you try to sleep the more awake you become, and so it is a vicious circle. There are a few simple steps you can take to fall asleep, but if you find that you regularly cannot sleep try and analyse why. Is there some problem nagging away that needs to be sorted out? Often the problem is that your body does not really need as much sleep as you think it does and so it stays awake. Perhaps the problem is trying to get too much sleep!

Have a good night's sleep. If you really don't feel tired, then the answer is don't go to bed. Stay up and watch the late night film, or read a book, write the letters that you've been meaning to answer for so long, in fact anything rather than go to bed. Once you start to occupy your mind you may feel tired and ready to sleep. If not, then stay up until you begin to feel reasonably tired. Your body won't let you stay up a whole night, so don't worry! Probably after one or two late nights you will find that you begin to sleep better. If your body gets into the habit of going to bed a little later, and perhaps even waking up earlier, you will discover that your sleep will become much deeper and you will feel much more refreshed in the morning. There really is nothing more satisfying than waking up after a really deep sleep and feeling totally relaxed and at peace with the world, ready to face whatever the day may bring.

The secret of a good night's sleep is learning how to relax. One of the most relaxing ways to end the day is to soak in a warm bath and just let your muscles unwind naturally. Add some of your favourite bubble bath or herbal salts too to make your bath really enjoyable.

Have a hot milky drink like cocoa, try and avoid coffee as this is a stimulant and will keep you awake. There are several herbal drinks on the market that have been tried through the ages. These are considered *natural* sleep inducers, and are non-habit forming.

Your body loves routine of any kind and will soon regulate itself to any routine that suits your lifestyle. Whether it is getting up at four o'clock each morning because you are a postman, or not getting to bed until two o'clock because you work in the theatre, whatever your routine your body will adjust to it, just as long as you are getting sufficient sleep. It does not matter so much *when* you sleep, as long as you get *enough*. So whatever your occupation or lifestyle, try and get into a routine at night and go to bed at the same time, bath at the same time, have your last drink, put the lights out and put the dog to bed, all at the same time each night and you will find that your body will quickly get used to this and be prepared to go to sleep at night.

If you have difficulty sleeping then find out whether or not exercise would be good for you at night. Some people find that a ten minute exercise routine, followed by a relaxation exercise, helps them sleep like a log. Other people find it much too stimulating and prefer to exercise in the morning to get them ready for the day. This is merely a matter of personal preference. Maybe you would like some exercise at night but cannot face a set fitness routine before going to bed, so instead go for a stroll around the block, or take the dog for a short walk. It might just relieve any tension and help you sleep more soundly.

If you are one of these people who can nod off in a chair after lunch or take a short nap whilst watching television, but cannot sleep at night, then avoid sleeping during the day however tired you may be. It won't be long before you no longer need your afternoon snooze and begin to sleep at night.

Try and bring your evening to a relaxing close. Sit and unwind with your bedtime drink, listen to some relaxing music, or just lie back and let your thoughts take over. Clock radios are often beneficial to have beside your bed because they switch themselves on and off, so you can lie in bed and relax to your favourite late night radio programme. If you fall asleep whilst it is on it will not matter because the radio will switch itself off.

Above all, don't worry about not sleeping as this will only keep you awake. Don't start taking sleeping pills, but learn to relax and if you get into a nightly sleeping pattern you will find all will be well. Don't count sheep as this will only serve to stimulate the brain too, and at three o'clock in the morning when over five thousand sheep have jumped the fence you will still be as wide awake as ever. If you get to bed and find you cannot sleep, then read a novel or start writing your thoughts down on paper, it doesn't matter what they are but you might find it very therapeutic. Sleep will come eventually, and if you have a bad night, tomorrow night will be better. If your body needs sleep it will soon tell you, so have a good night!

Chapter Twelve

Your Physical Appearance

Looking after your body and keeping fit does not only mean having a strong constitution and carefully exercising your muscles, but it means looking physically fit too. Physical appearance is far more than vanity; if you look good then you feel good too. Looking after your skin, hair, teeth, and nails is just as important to your general fitness as looking after your limbs and muscles.

Obviously *how* you look will depend a great deal on how you treat your body. As we said before, we are what we eat, and if you eat the wrong things, abuse the body with heavy drinking and smoking, and lack essential nutrients, then this will be reflected in your physical appearance. Apart from making you appear healthy, correct attention to your physical appearance will keep you looking youthful. If you abuse your body then it will abuse you by making you look old before your time.

In our present age, how we look is very important to both men and women, and it is just as necessary for men as well as women to look after their skin and hair and keep it in peak condition. It seems that men are becoming much more aware of their physical appearance and are going to much greater lengths to keep it right. The following advice is applicable to both men and women alike. Let us look first at what is sometimes called the largest bodily organ, the skin.

Skin

The skin is something that we generally take very much for granted, it covers our whole body and as long as it is kept clean, smells nice, and has no unusual rashes or spots we don't take any notice of it. What, however, is going on inside the body is often shown on the outside. The skin is more than just a covering to the body. It is generally about 16% of our total bodily weight and covers an area of approximately twenty square feet – which is a large area when you think of how much wall-paper you would need to cover a wall that size. Now you know why fat people are said to be 'as big as a house'!

The skin is very elastic and is made up of several different layers:

1   The epidermis – made up mostly of dead cells which act as a waterproof protective barrier. This layer is constantly being rubbed off by our clothes, towels, and so on. Immediately underneath the dead skin is a layer of living cells which replace the skin we rub off.

2   The dermis – contains the sweat glands, hair roots and the nerves of our skin, which give us the sense of touch and pain. Also many hundreds of blood vessels to keep the skin nourished and in good condition.

3   Subcutaneous fatty layer – any excess fat on the body is stored under the skin.

The skin is very complex in structure and is approximately one to two millimetres thick, although much thinner in areas such as the eyelids. Its main function is to protect us from harmful bacteria and physical damage. It is a sensory organ so that we are able to feel sensations such as pain and heat , and so it provides an information service to our brain. The skin can also absorb the sun's rays which contain Vitamin D. The blood vessels in the skin are important to the control of heat. They rise to the surface when we are very hot, and you will notice this particularly in your hands on a very hot day when the veins rise to the surface. On a cold day they contract to keep the body warm and preserve energy. The skin also acts to control heat by containing millions of sweat glands through which we lose water – perspiration.

Our skin plays a very valuable part in our lives and for us to remain healthy it must be looked after correctly, especially since as we become older it loses its elastic qualities and so becomes wrinkled and sagging. Exposure to sunlight can cause premature aging, and although the sun is beneficial to the body in small quantities, too much can be very harmful and at its worst can cause skin cancer. Skin cancer is prevalent in people who work constantly out of doors. If neglected, skin cancers can spread, but if looked after in the early stages can be totally cured.

Cigarettes too can damage the skin because they restrict Vitamin C to the body which is necessary for a clear and healthy skin. Cigarettes are another cause of premature aging.

Look after your body by giving up smoking, and paying particular attention to your diet. Fruit and fresh vegetables will keep your skin looking radiant. Keep it soft and supple by applying a moisturising cream, especially if your skin is going to be exposed to the elements. Men should apply cream after shaving and this will prevent it from becoming dry.

Obviously washing is important to keep the pores clean and the body free from dirt. However excessive washing can dry up the skin and remove natural oils from the body so be sparing with the soap except in places where you perspire heavily, such as under the arms. Perspiration is always considered to be offensive and a nuisance, but it is in fact a necessary function. It rids the body of waste products and bacteria through the three million pores in the skin and regular washing and attention to cleanliness will get rid of any body odour. Deodorants are available but some can block the pores and irritate the skin so care should be taken in their application, and never use them on skin that is broken or already irritated. Nothing can take the place of regular washing.

Women should take particular care to remove every trace of make-up at night and cleanse the skin thoroughly to remove any traces of dirt which clogs the pores. Apply a moisturiser before applying any make-up as this will build up a protective barrier and prevent the skin from becoming dry. If you look after your skin, not only what goes on it but what goes inside too, and suitably protect it from the sun, wind and rain, then you should not have any problems and will glow with health.

Problems

ACNE – This often causes problems during the years of puberty when an excess amount of sebum is produced by the sebaceous glands. Inflamed spots appear on the face, neck, and back, which are painful and can leave scars. Unfortunately there is no cure and it is a problem that adolescents have to cope with in the knowledge that they will grow out of it. The condition can, however, be improved by careful use of antiseptic soaps and medicated creams and lotions that are now on the market. Sunray treatment can be helpful in some cases as it dries up the skin and makes it peel. Some doctors believe that acne is aggravated by certain food substances, such as chocolate, although there is no concrete proof of this. If you do suffer from acne it might be worth making a note of all that you eat and noting if the condition seems worse after having eaten a particular product.

ATHLETE'S FOOT – This is a fungus infection that occurs between the toes (and sometimes the soles) and results in painful flaking skin that is aggravated by perspiration. It is important, therefore, to keep the feet clean, cool and dry by using talcum powder or special athlete's foot powder that is available from most chemists. It is infectious so it is necessary to avoid public places, such as swimming baths, where it is likely to be passed on. Clean socks and stockings daily are a must.

BLACKHEADS – These are small plugs of oil or dirt that block the pores. They are not painful but look unsightly. They can be removed gently by using a hot flannel as a compress and rubbing briskly to open the pores and removing the dirt.

BOILS – These are sweat glands that become infected and rise up into painful bumps, often with a slight discharge. They can appear when a person is feeling very low, or can be caused by friction, such as the rubbing of a shirt collar. There is no need to seek medical advice unless a large number occur suddenly or they are very painful. They will heal themselves in time.

BROKEN VEINS – These can appear anywhere on the body, especially on the face, where the capillaries are very fragile and can only be removed professionally with an electronic needle. They can be escaped by avoiding extremes in temperature and making sure you have sufficient Vitamin C in your diet.

BRUISES – These occur after a heavy blow to the skin causing blood vessels to break. Blood seeps under the skin, appearing blue from the surface, and eventually yellow as it heals and then disappears. Some people bruise more easily than others, but it is not usually serious.

COLD SORES – These are caused by a virus and appear as painful red lumps anywhere on the body, but particularly around the mouth. They can be painful but not serious, and can be relieved by rubbing on some antiseptic cream.

DERMATITIS – This is the name given to inflammation and flaking of the skin, normally caused by an allergy of some kind. It is the general term given to psoriasis and eczema. Often the cause is unknown but it can result from an emotional upset, contact with chemicals such as detergent, or an allergy to a particular food substance. The skin becomes red and scaly and gradually peels off. If a cause is identified then it can be prevented in future, but if it is a nervous condition then there really is no prevention. The condition can be relieved by special ointments and creams. In very bad cases there are drugs available that will slow down the growth rate of the epidermis cells, but this is only in very extreme cases.

HIVES – An allergic disorder caused by pollen, food,or

drugs and results in large red swollen patches. The body releases a chemical called histamine which causes blood vessels to swell. Can be treated by creams and antihistamine tablets, and is not serious unless the swelling occurs around the mouth or throat and interferes with breathing.

MOLES – These are small brown, harmless marks that can occur anywhere on the body. Some people call them beauty spots. They can be removed surgically but no attempt should ever be made to remove them yourself.

WARTS – These are growths that appear on the skin. They are caused by a virus and are perfectly harmless and will eventually disappear on their own. They sometimes respond to chemicals or to 'freezing'.

Looking After Your Face

Although all your skin needs looking after, your face is particularly important for that is what people see, and your face, more than anything, has an unkind habit of showing your age if you don't treat it properly

Abrasive soaps remove layers of dead skin and keep the face glowing and bright, so buy soaps that contain oatmeal, or rub the skin with an oatmeal mixture once a week. Removing dead skin is said to stimulate cell production and new healthy cells keep you looking fresh and young. Men shave daily and so already remove a layer of skin and this helps them keep a soft skin.

The circulation can be stimulated by splashing your face with ice cold water, this will tighten up the skin and keep it fresh.

Give yourself a home facial sauna by pouring some boiling water into a bowl on top of a few mint leaves or flower petals. Place your face over the bowl with a towel over your head and let the steam open up your pores and deep cleanse your face for a few minutes. After your mini sauna splash your face with cold water and pat it dry with a towel. Your skin will feel tingling and alive.

131

If your skin has a tendency to be dry, then always use a moisturiser and a sun barrier cream when braving the elements. Men should try and use an oil based after-shave rather than an alcohol-based one which can have a drying effect on the skin. You will also find that oil based perfumes and after-shave lotions will retain their fragrance for a lot longer too.

Teeth. The major function of teeth, of course, is to bite and chew, but there is a lot to be said for clean and healthy teeth when considering a person's physical appearance. Our teeth are not easy to keep clean and unlike rabbit's teeth they do not keep growing when they get worn.

Tooth decay is one of the most common disorders in humans today, probably because we eat too many sweet foods which cause it. The enamel is slowly destroyed and a cavity is formed; if this is not filled in time the whole tooth will become rotten and will cause toothache. Careful brushing at least twice daily is essential to healthy teeth, but never neglect the gums as many teeth (and healthy teeth too) are lost through gum disease, so be sure to clean the area where the gum meets the teeth. Dental cleanliness was drummed into us all at school, but it is just as important for adults. Don't have a toothbrush that is too hard as this could damage your gums. One that is too soft could be ineffective and leave particles of food behind that will encourage bacteria. Whether you have a nylon or a bristle brush is purely a matter of taste, (no pun intended!) but nylon is generally thought to be preferable.

With regular brushing, six monthly visits to your dentist should be all you require to maintain strong and healthy teeth and gums. There is no reason why you should ever require false teeth if you look after your own. So give everyone an attractive smile today.

Eyes. As with teeth it is vital to have these checked regularly. Contact lenses now improve the appearance if you do have to wear glasses permanently. Your eyes are in fact muscles, so it is necessary to keep them strong and well rested.

Whatever you are doing make sure that you have enough light as eyes can easily be weakened by poor light. If your eyes are tired then refresh them by splashing the lids with cold water or lie down with a couple of cotton wool pads soaked in cold water on your eyes and relax.

Never rub your eyes as this can lead to infection. If something such as a particle of dust goes into your eye then let it come out on its own by blinking. Rubbing your eyes will make it go in further and could scratch your eyeball. Blinking will stimulate the tear ducts and the foreign body will soon come out.

Inflammation of the eye is called conjunctivitis and can be caused by an infection or a foreign body, perhaps an ingrowing eyelash. If your eyes are sore be sure to seek medical advice straightaway. Eyes can be protected by dark glasses and if they are sore can be bathed with a solution of warm water, or a medical lotion. Infection can cause a stye to occur on the eyelid, but this will go of its own accord and can be eased by bathing the infected eye. If you ever bathe both eyes, always use a new and separate piece of cotton wool for each eye, otherwise infection could spread.

Our eyes are wonderful organs and we should always be thankful for good eyesight. As with so many things we never fully appreciate it as we should. If you take care not to strain your eyes, always have sufficient light to work by, and plenty of sleep, your eyes should remain strong and bright.

Hair Care. Hair is found all over the body, protecting it, and keeping it warm. The root of the hair is alive, although the hair itself is made up of dead cells. We lose up to a hundred each day, but don't worry since at any one time a full head of hair has approximately 150,000 hairs. The thickness and texture is inherited from your parents.

Hair is made out of Keratin and is in three layers:

1   Medulla – a hollow central core.
2   Cortex – this gives the hair its colour.
3   Cuticle – an outer covering of the hair.

The condition of your hair depends not only on what you do to the hair itself, but, as always, upon what you eat. If you are in good general health, then your hair will be too. Vitamin B is essential to strong healthy hair as are proteins, for hair itself is a type of protein.

To improve the physical appearance of your hair, conditioners will make the cuticle lie smooth and flat so that it reflects the light and so your hair will shine. We wash it to make it look good rather than for health reasons, although clean hair is important for the condition of our scalp.

If you have oily hair wash it at least twice a week and try and eat fewer greasy foods, especially fried food.

If your hair is dry then wash it less frequently, but at least once a week, and use a conditioner. Use an appropriate shampoo for your hair, and try occasionally massaging an oil treatment into your hair. You can make one yourself by mixing an egg with some oil and vinegar. Leave it on your hair for five to ten minutes and then shampoo it.

Dry as well as greasy hair can result in dandruff. If you do have dandruff, use an appropriate shampoo, brush daily to stimulate the blood supply, and wear it in a shorter style if possible. Always make sure that your brushes and combs are perfectly clean as dirt can lead to infection.

Always avoid pulling at your hair when it is wet, and comb it as little as possible for wet hair is weak and the ends can easily split. If you do have any hair or scalp problems it is advisable to visit your doctor. It may be that your shampoo is too harsh and is removing the essential natural oils.

Hair Loss. Baldness in men is a constant source of worry to many. One in five men in Britain goes at least partially bald, and if it is hereditary then there simply is no solution. Sorry! If your hair's going to fall out, it will. Hair can, of course, be lost due to mental strain, illness and skin ailments, but if it is part of your body's inheritance then nothing can be done to slow down or stop hair loss, except castration – which is rather a drastic way to keep your hair!

Every day we lose a certain number of hairs, but these are replaced. This means that over a period of about three years we get a completely new head of hair. In a balding man these hairs are either not replaced, or else grow much finer in texture until he eventually becomes bald, or partially bald.

If you look after your hair and make sure that it is not too dry and brittle or even greasy then there is no reason why it should fall out too quickly. It won't fall out over night anyway! Keep yourself in good condition too, because hair will fall out quicker if you are in poor health, and don't worry about hair loss, it is perfectly natural and worry might make it fall out even faster!

Don't try and disguise baldness by combing hair from the back or a few straggly bits across the top, it looks awful and it is painfully obvious what you are trying to do. Some men look good with bald heads anyway. If you really hate being bald then there are methods of disguising the fact, although don't be taken in by people offering massage, potions, manure, or anything else to make your hair grow. It won't, and if anyone had a miracle cure he would soon be a millionaire. More satisfactory methods are:

* Toupees – wigs and toupees have improved tremendously over the past few years and are now within the price range of most people. It is generally advisable today to buy a man-made fibre wig. You will find that you will get a better colour match (a poor match will give you away immediately), it will be much easier to look after, and it won't fade in the sun. There are a variety of bases available too that are light and let your head breathe. If you intend to wear a toupee permanently then invest in two as a safety precaution – it would be awful if you spilt paint on one and had to go to work bald the next day!

* Hair weaving – In this method hair is attached by weaving hair from one side of the bald patch to the other. It can look good but has the disadvantage of being attached

to your own hair so that as your hair grows the weave becomes loose and therefore needs to be re-fitted every month to six weeks. Much more expensive than a toupee, and difficult to wash as the weave can become tangled.

* Transplants – This technique is becoming far more widely used and is improving all the time. Hair is taken from the back of your head and planted on the bald areas. A lengthy process as each hair root has to be transplanted. It is, therefore, a very lengthy procedure, and quite painful too. Unfortunately there are no real guarantees that the hair will grow. So, serious thought must be given before such a course of treatment is embarked upon. Always consult a reputable clinic.

Obviously there is nothing like having your own hair, so treat what you have got with respect. Remember that there is nothing wrong with a bald head, it can look very masculine and need not be a sign of old age. Youngsters these days have their heads shaved! But if you feel better having hair and think it makes you look better, and you feel psychologically happier then go *ahead* and replace what nature has taken away from you.

Hand it to Yourself. In both men and women it is essential to think about your hands. Usually we take our hands for granted and yet we use them so very much. When you meet someone for the first time, what do you do? Yes, you shake hands. That hand says a lot about you, and there's nothing worse than shaking a rough and coarse skinned hand. If you want to describe something, you do it with your hands, for besides being practical they also express your individual personality.

Each hand has twenty-eight bones, making it very flexible. The hand is one of the most sensitive parts of the body. They become the 'eyes' of a blind person, and once you have damaged them and let them get out of condition you will find it very difficult to return to the original condition. Whenever possible, protect your hands by wearing gloves. Rubber gloves if you are using chemicals or abrasives, leather gloves if you are in the garden pruning roses, and warm gloves if the weather is cold.

Use hand creams to stop them getting dry, and keep them scrupulously clean too because the hand that feeds you could so easily be the hand that poisons you by spreading bacteria and infections.

Don't neglect your fingernails either. Nails are very similar to hair because they are made of keratin. Like hair they will reflect your general health by becoming brittle if below par. Your nails grow approximately one-and-a-half inches a year, but faster if you use the tips of your fingers a great deal, if you are a typist for example.

When filing your nails it is better to use an emery board than a harsh metal file. Keep your nails carefully cut and clean so that they don't cause infection. Make sure the cuticle can be seen and use creams on your fingers around the nails to keep the skin soft. Take care not to scratch or damage the nail as it will take several months for it to grow out.

Changing Your Appearance

I wonder how many people are really happy with their physical appearance? Have you ever thought that your nose is too big, or your chin looks wrong? Few people are truly satisfied, and if your physical appearance causes you great emotional distress then today there is the possibility of plastic surgery.

Plastic surgery can be very expensive and is usually only performed under the National Health in cases of extreme medical defect, perhaps after a severe facial burn or to improve breathing after a broken nose. Cosmetic surgery is performed only after very careful consideration and then only under the advice of a doctor. On the whole it is much better to stick to the face nature gave you. Surgery can, however, straighten noses, alter the shape of noses and chins, remove bags from under eyes, pull in ears that stick out, and so on.

Unfortunately the healing process takes time, usually six months or more, whatever the operation, and very often the patient is disappointed with the result. A surgeon can only use what you have in the first place, he cannot give you a nose like a film star of your choice. No-one can know the result until several months after the operation when swelling and bruising disappear. So, plastic surgery is not something to be gone into lightly, and is only advisable in very special cases.

General Guide to Looking Good

Looking good means caring about your physical appearance. It is everyone's right to make the very best of what he has, for how you will look will reflect to other people the kind of person you really are. If you look untidy and a mess then that is how your lifestyle is going to appear to other people. If you don't respect your own appearance then people will not respect you as a person. So, here's how to improve your general appearance:

* First, make certain that you are in good physical condition. Check your diet and your weight to make sure you are eating the correct foods, plenty of fresh vegetables and fruit will give you a clear and healthy looking skin. Stop smoking. This will make you look and feel better, and won't make you socially unacceptable by smelling of stale tobacco. Get plenty of exercise.

* Pay attention to personal cleanliness. Perhaps your friends are too polite to tell you that you have BO. Change your clothes daily. Pamper yourself by buying nice scented soaps, and your favourite perfume or after shave, but don't overdo it. A nice subtle fragrance of cologne is far more acceptable than a strong scent that knocks everyone backwards each time you enter the room. Even the most expensive perfumes can smell like air fresheners in excess.

* Look after your hair. Don't let it get too greasy. Choose a style that suits you and is easy to manage. Don't make the mistake of thinking long flowing hair will make

you look youthful. Older people with long hair often look twice their age, so get your best friend to be honest and tell you if your hair style really suits you.

* Take pride in your dress. Don't look sloppy or untidy, and this again will reflect on you as a person. This does not mean going to extremes and looking as if you are going to a wedding every day of the week, but it does mean that whatever unexpected situation may occur you will be ready for it and not feel too untidy.

* Learn how to relax fully at the end of each day. A relaxed and carefree nature will soon change your appearance. If you remain too tense you will age prematurely, even go grey prematurely. If you are relaxed you will not only feel better yourself, but will find that you are in a better frame of mind to face the day. You will become a much nicer you.

So, go to a full-length mirror and have a good long hard look at yourself NOW. Do you like what you see? If not, it's never too late to do something about it.

Chapter Thirteen

Tension and Bad Posture

All of us get backache sometimes. Usually it is because too much strain has been put on the backbone, bending it out of its natural shape. This strain comes because none of us thinks about our back in every day life until it starts to cause us some trouble. Then it may be too late. Once you get into bad habits your posture becomes bad and then you constantly get backache, for good posture means preserving the natural shape of your back as closely as possible, whatever you are doing. Bad posture means that whatever you are doing your spine will be the wrong shape, it will be taking a lot more strain than it needs to and will give you trouble.

Bad posture does not only mean a bad back either, it can result in poor breathing, depression, leg ache, and tired muscles. If you stand tall and erect with your head held high you will have a feeling of well-being too. It affects how you look, how you walk, how you sit and even how tall you look.

Poor posture can be a result of many things, it could be that you are overweight or simply that you have mistreated your back, not paid attention to how you walk and over the years have begun to slouch. At all times try and keep your head up and your shoulders straight and the lower part of your back hollow. Not only will you feel better, but you will look better too.

Your spine is a complex structure of bones, muscle and cartilage. The spine is made up of a column of vertebrae with cushions of cartilage in between that act as shock absorbers. When the posture is bad the vertebrae begin to protrude slightly and so cause pain if any kind of strain is put upon them. When the posture is correct you can move at will without pain or damage.

The causes of bad posture are constant misuse. For example, how do you bend to pick something up? The correct way is to bend from the knees, not from the waist. Bending from the waist makes the back curved.

If you have to lift something heavy bend your knees and make the legs do the work, not your back. If you have bad posture and strain to lift something the strain will be much worse. One of the worst things you can carry is your own fat. If you are overweight you are putting a strain on your back *all the time*. If you do have back trouble try and lose some weight. For example, if you are half a stone overweight, think how your back would feel carrying half a stone of potatoes around every day!

Many modern shoes today with high heels and platforms cause bad posture by making you walk awkwardly. By all means be fashionable, but not at the expense of your back. Stiletto heels may make your legs look fantastic, but who's going to look at your legs if you are round shouldered and walk badly. The person who walks into a room with head held high and spine straight will turn far more heads.

Good posture means a straight pelvis, spine in a natural curve, abdomen in and chest out. Years ago people used to think walking around in a military style was good for the posture, with the shoulders forced back. Forcing muscles, however, causes tension, and tension leads to bad posture. During the day, try and avoid tension as much as possible. If you learn to relax in your spare moments, and not get irritated over silly little things that you can do nothing about you will find that you are far less tense.

The way to achieve good posture is to imagine that you are suspended from the ceiling by a cord that passes through your head and down your spine to your pelvis. By standing straight like this your body will find the correct balance and your posture will be good. Learn how to support your weight too, resting it equally on both feet. If you stand on one foot, or rest on one foot, there will be an unequal distribution of weight, resulting in one thing – bad posture.

If your posture is bad, and a high percentage of the population is round shouldered, it is worth doing something about it NOW. It certainly will not improve on its own, and is likely to get worse as you get older.

First, look at how you stand. Do you tend to stoop? This may be caused by washing up at a low sink unit, or working at a low desk where you have to bend your shoulders. If you do stoop, bend your knees rather than your shoulders when you have to bring yourself down to a certain height. If it is essential that you bend over a desk to work, then straighten yourself up every so often and put your hands behind your head and have a good stretch.

When sitting, make sure that the chair has a high back so that it supports you. Unless it is perfectly placed a low-backed chair can only cut into the middle of your back and will offer you no support. Take note too how you actually sit down. Do you simply slump back in a chair? If so try lowering yourself into it by bending your knees and keeping your spine straight. If possible hold your work in the air nearer your head, rather then bending your head down to look at it. This again will strengthen the back tremendously.

If you have to carry something heavy, perhaps a brief case or a bag of shopping, try and distribute the weight evenly so that it is not continually on one side. If you can, carry two bags of equal weight so that there is the same amount of strain on each shoulder. If you cannot do this then frequently change the bag from hand to hand every few minutes so that each shoulder bears the weight for an equal length of time.

Finally, make a good check of your bed. This could be the root cause of your back trouble and bad posture. A bed that is too soft will curve your spine and cause unnecessary tension. A firm mattress will support the spine and keep it naturally straight. You may try putting a piece of hardboard under the mattress if you cannot afford to buy a firm one, this will have just the same effect. You might find it difficult to sleep on at first, but once you get used to it your back will be much better for it. It's better to have a couple of uncomfortable nights and end up with perfect posture than to sleep on a soft and worn out mattress and have backache for the rest of your life. You will move, feel, and look better too, so hold your head up high and regain the posture nature gave you.

Chapter Fourteen

Simple Massage

One of the most relaxing ways of toning up your muscles and relieving tension in the body is by massage and manipulation of the body. Unfortunately the art of massage is sadly neglected and conjures up a picture of a strong muscular masseur in a steamy sauna bath. There is, however, no reason at all why you should not massage yourself, or get your husband or wife to do it for you. It is so easy and can be soothing and relaxing not only for the person being massaged, but also the person doing it.

There are many books available on massage and you might like to dip into them when you are next in your local public library. But don't feel that you have to learn very special techniques, you will find that it comes quite naturally and you will soon discover which movements are the most relaxing.

The best time to be massaged is straight after having a bath, but make sure that it is done in a warm room so that you don't get cold. If you are going to massage someone you will first need some oil. There are many on the market that vary in price, but the cheapest and just as effective is ordinary baby oil. The oil will keep your hands soft and supple and keep your movements smooth and relaxing.

Start in the areas where tension builds up, at the neck and shoulders, moving your hands firmly but gently in a circular motion. Put a hand on each shoulder blade and massage the neck and between the shoulders with your thumbs. Gradually work your way down the body, concentrating on the spine, and don't be afraid to put on too much pressure. Move your way up and down the sides of the spine, and pay particular attention to the small of the back. Grasp your hands around the top of the pelvis and massage the spine on either side with your finger tips, gently squeezing the body between your thumb and finger tips at the same time.

Work your way all over the back, experiment with different movements. Rub your finger tips in a circular motion, kneed the back with your knuckles, push down with the palms of your hands, and so on. The oil will help you to keep your movements smooth, and you will soon discover that the movements become quite natural after a time. Learn how to squeeze the skin and muscles to release the tension, and don't forget the arms, legs and feet either, they all benefit from a good massage.

If you don't have anyone to massage you, don't despair! Using your baby oil, simply smooth it over your body and massage yourself. Again start at the neck with both hands, then massage one shoulder at a time, your right shoulder with your left hand, then your left shoulder with your right hand. Massage your spine, you will find the various movements and degrees of pressure will come perfectly naturally, and pay particular attention to your feet, rubbing oil between your toes and massaging them in a circular motion. You will find that it removes tension and keeps your limbs supple, your skin soft, and your body totally relaxed.

Massaging the Scalp. Massage of the scalp will stimulate the blood flow and so keep your hair healthier and in better condition. Simply push your fingers into your hair and move your fingers in a circular motion. You will find that if you raise and lower your eye-brows at the same time this will increase the effect. After about five minutes massage, making sure you cover the back and sides of your head too, place your thumbs on your temples and your fingers on the top of your head. Pushing firmly, wiggle your thumbs up and down so that your scalp moves up and down. Finally, push your fingers into your hair and close them up together so that hair is trapped between each finger. Give a very gentle tug, not too hard, just a couple of times, and this again will increase the blood flow to the roots of your hair.

Massage Your Face. To keep the skin soft and supple on your face, don't forget to massage this too. First, begin with the forehead. Push the palm of your hand flat against it and start by raising your eyebrows up and down, pushing as hard as you can with your palm. Now, place your thumbs just above your ears and your fingertips on your forehead and push your finger tips together so that it pushes the skin on your forehead from side to side. Finally, relax the forehead altogether and with your left hand stroke your forehead gently from right temple to left temple ten times, and then repeat with the other hand. Concentrate on your forehead at the same time and imagine any wrinkles being ironed out by your hand. Gentle stroking of the forehead can be very relaxing, and is a technique often used by mothers to send their babies to sleep, simply by gently stroking their forehead.

Now massage your cheeks by placing the palms of your hands on each cheek and gently move them round in a circular movement. Purse your lips as though you were going to whistle and lightly stroke your cheeks with your finger tips.

Massage the mouth and chin by closing your mouth, raising your chin and gently move your fingertips (which should be pressed together) over your throat up to your chin, over the chin to the mouth, and at the mouth pull your hands apart so that the finger tips go across your mouth, cheeks and eventually touch your ears. Always stroke from your throat to your mouth, not the other way round; the movement means making a letter 'T' with your fingers, your throat being the base and your ears at each side of the top. It sounds complicated, but if you aim to cover the area as if the letter 'T' had been painted on the lower half of your face you will find it quite easy.

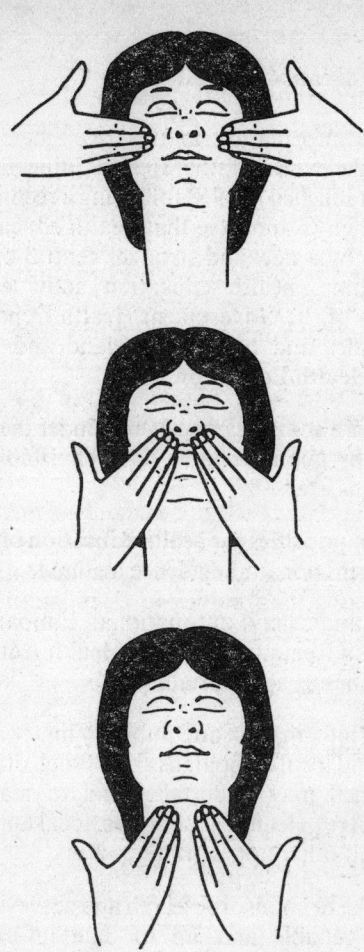

Ending the day with a nice gentle massage will relieve the body of all the tension that has built up over the day. The relaxing, rhythmical movements will remove your aches and pains, and pave the way for a restful and refreshing sleep, so that when you wake up in the morning you really will feel fit for life.

The Health Education Council

Much of the information in this book has been based directly on the work of the Health Education Council which was established in 1968 following a recommendation from the Cohen Committee that health education should be promoted by a new and stronger central organisation. Until that time, health education activities were the responsibility of the Government Health Departments for England, Wales and Northern Ireland and the Central Council for Health Education.

The Council is a company, registered under the Companies Act, limited by guarantee and given charitable status. Its main functions are:

*To advise on priorities for health education on the basis of the best information and evidence available.

*To devise and carry out national campaigns, in co-operation with Regional and Area Health Authorities and local authorities as appropriate.

*To produce information and publicity material in support of national and local campaigns and of such other activities as the Council may undertake; and to make material available to Area Health Authorities, local authorities and voluntary and other appropriate bodies.

*To undertake or sponsor research and surveys designed to ensure that reliable and up to date information and statistics are available on which to base the campaigns and other activities of the Council.

*To seek advice and to review relevant medical, epi-dermiological, sociological. psychological and other information available and, as necessary to undertake or sponsor research and surveys designed to obtain such information, to assist the Council in its determination of priorities and in the measurement of the effectiveness of the results of its national and experimental campaigns.

*To act as the national centre of expertise and knowledge in all aspects of health education, so that advice is available at all times to Area Health Authorities and others engaged in health education; and, with the agreement of National Health Service and local authorities, educational and voluntary bodies, to co-ordinate health education activities where appropriate.

*To encourage and promote training in health education work; and to provide to other bodies advice and guidance on the organisation and content of courses of training, together with such practical help as may seem appropriate and within the resources of the Council.

*To co-operate with local education authorities, educational establishments and the School's Council in the development of health education in schools, colleges and polytechnics.

*To maintain contact with national voluntary bodies engaged in particular aspects of health education work; and to give aid and advice to such bodies.

*To publish material of interest and value to those engaged in health education.

Publications

The Council produces a wide range of publications – posters, leaflets and books – dealing with many aspects of health care. These are distributed in bulk to the health education sections of Area Health Authorities, where they are available to the general public. Personal callers can select publications of interest from a display at the Council's London headquarters. Most of them are free of charge.

Among the topics covered are:
alcoholism, smoking, use of the NHS, self-treatment, health in middle age, care of the elderly, hyperthermia, breast self-examination, child welfare and parentcraft, dental health, foot health, home safety, safe use of medicines, food hygiene, influenza, scabies, measles, rubella, exercise, diet, drugs, the menopause, cystitis, helping the deaf, nutrition, breast feeding, personal hygiene, sex education, family planning, sexually transmitted infections.

The Council also publishes a bi-monthly newspaper (Health Education News) and a quarterly professional journal (Health Education Journal). The Council also provides a subscription service which provides subscribers with publications, copies of new leaflets and posters as they come out, and other information of interest to health education.

Addresses

Health Education Council (covers England, Wales, N. Ireland) 78 New Oxford Street, London WC1A 1AH. Tel: 01-637 1881
Scottish Health Education Unit, 21 Lansdowne Crescent, Edinburgh, EH12 5EH. Tel: 031-337 3251
Sports Council (England) 70 Brompton Road, London SW3 1EX. Tel: 01-589 3411
Sports Council for Wales, National Sports Centre, Sophia Gardens, Cardiff, Tel: 0222-397 571
Scottish Sports Council, 1 St. Colme Street, Edinburgh, EH3 6AA. Tel: 031-225 8411
Sports Council for Northern Ireland, 49 Malone Road, Belfast BT9 6RZ, Tel: 0232-663 154